GET FIT

not fat

**150 ways to build
fitness into your life**

Greg Whyte

Kyle Cathie Limited

'To my Channel-swimming girls: anything is possible!'

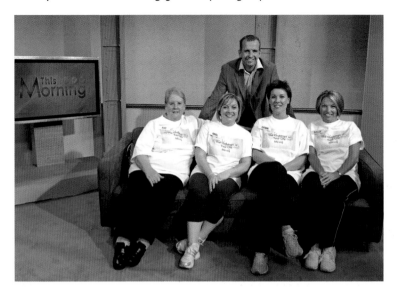

First published in Great Britain in 2008 by
Kyle Cathie Limited
www.kylecathie.com

10 9 8 7 6 5 4 3 2 1

ISBN 978-1-85626-786-1

Text © 2008 Greg Whyte
Photography © 2008 Tony Chau
(see additional acknowledgements on page 192)
Book design © 2008 Kyle Cathie Limited

Project editor: Jennifer Wheatley
Designer: Alison Fenton
Photographer: Tony Chau (see also page 192)
Copy editor: Stephanie Evans
Editorial assistant: Vicki Murrell
Production Director: Sha Huxtable

A Cataloguing In Publication record for this title is available
from the British Library.

Printed in China

contents

Foreword by David Walliams

A week after I swam the Channel, I gave Greg a watch as a thank-you present. On the back of the watch I had had engraved 'We did it!' and the date I completed my crossing, 4 July 2006. Comic Relief set up a meeting with Professor Greg Whyte a year before my Channel crossing attempt. After meeting my comedy partner Matt Lucas, meeting Greg was the most fortunate meeting of my life. He single-handedly helped me achieve something that I had foolishly suggested to do on a trip to Ethiopia, a proposition that became more terrifying the more I found out about it.

Greg proved to be a huge fountain of knowledge about every aspect of sport and fitness: the physical aspects, of course, but the mental aspects too. Previously I had swum only a mile in a pool, rather than 25 miles in the sea. He drove me to an absolute peak of fitness. At school I was the fat boy who always came last in the cross-country race, and I ended up winning an award at the Sports Personality of the Year!

Most important, Greg proved to be a great friend too. He treated me with great care and compassion as I undertook the most daunting challenge of my life. No one is better placed to write a book like this. Anyone wanting to improve their health and fitness will learn so much from Greg's intelligent and yet simple and straightforward advice. I did everything he told me to do, and I achieved the impossible. And when I had the words 'We did it' engraved on the watch, I really meant it. He was there for me every step of the way. He changed my life – maybe he can change yours too.

David Walliams

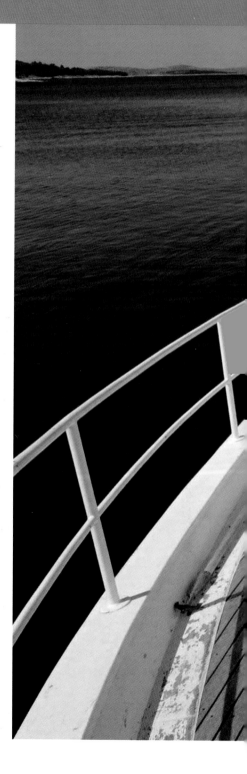

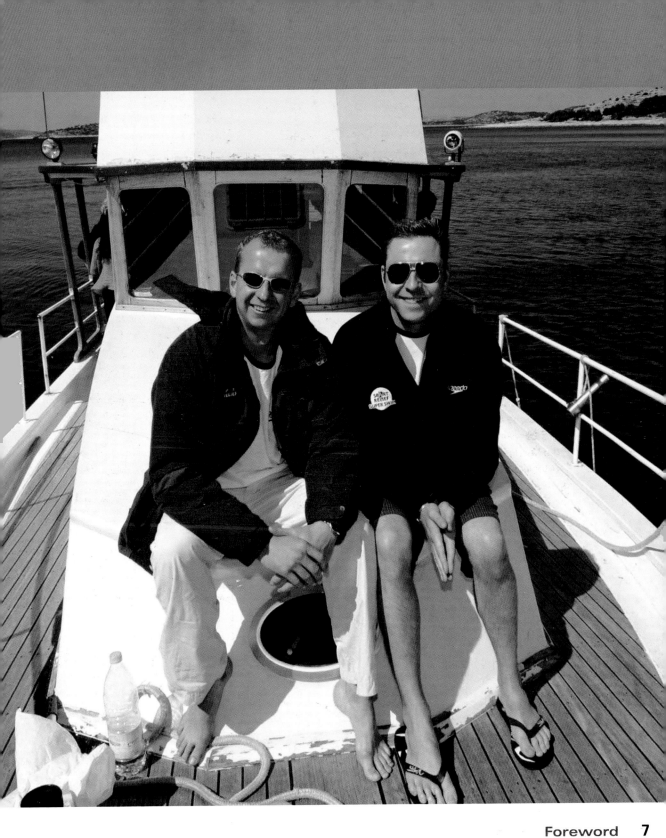

Fitness not fatness

I have been working in the field of health and fitness as an athlete, a sports scientist and a coach for more than two decades. During that time I have watched the obesity problem grow to become not only an epidemic in the UK, but a pandemic affecting all of Western society. Over that same period the focus in dealing with obesity has been almost entirely on reducing calorie consumption – dieting. The dieting phenomenon has been generated and perpetuated by an explosion of print, TV and electronic media attention on obesity and dieting. While I certainly endorse the importance of a healthy, balanced diet it is clear that the public has been misled into believing that dieting alone is the only weapon against fatness. Moreover, the diet message that bombards us daily often fails to recognise the dangers of excessive calorie restriction. Fad dieting associated with chronic calorie restriction can be as problematic as excessive calorie consumption. The quest of millions, mainly women, driven by the media, to achieve a sylph-like size 0 figure is often associated with a multitude of health problems. Furthermore, dieting alone rarely works in the long term as it often fails to result in a permanent change in body weight. Only 10 per cent of those who diet are able to maintain their weight loss in the long term. To put it another way, 90 per cent of those who diet to lose weight will constantly be on a diet!

Fat is an international issue

Despite the undeniable health benefits of exercise the developed world has become obsessed with fatness and diet. But why is fatness such an issue and is dieting the only way to conquer it? Obesity has become the focus of attention because it is the main visible sign of excessive calorie consumption and inactivity. Obesity is not a disease but a condition that leads to disease. It doubles the risk of heart disease and stroke and increases the risks of developing Type 2 diabetes and some cancers. In addition obesity leads to musculo-skeletal problems and disability and has negative psychological consequences, including depression and low self-esteem.

So why focus entirely on fatness? Although obesity is caused by several different factors, a gain in body weight as a result of an increase in fat mass (see page 18) is down to eating too many calories and exercising too little. Recent evidence suggests, however, that being obese is not in itself a health problem if you are physically fit. Burning off calories by way of exercise is receiving increased attention because of its sustained ability to control weight and its associated health benefits, such as better circulation, stronger immunity and higher mental and physical energy levels. There is indisputable evidence that regular exercise protects against chronic disease, most notably heart disease, diabetes and some forms of cancer – similar to the risks associated with obesity.

In light of the importance of physical activity for health, including weight management, and the seeming ineffectiveness of dieting alone, I felt it was time to put the spotlight on the importance of exercise and fitness. *Get Fit Not Fat* is part of a personal crusade to highlight the importance of physical activity and to make exercise accessible to everyone.

Fit for everyday life

Physical-activity recommendations from specialists in the field of exercise and health, including scientists, medics and government advisors, place an emphasis on moderate-intensity exercise for 30 minutes five times per week – equivalent to burning up 1,000 calories per week. We all know that exercise is good for us but most of us fail to meet this minimum guideline. There are two significant reasons for this inactivity: lack of facilities and perceived shortage of time for exercise, together with a lack of knowledge about what exercise to do, how hard to do it and for how long. The key to increasing levels of physical activity in the short term and maintaining it over time is to structure your exercise so that it both fits in with your lifestyle and is enjoyable. For the majority of us, the most acceptable and easiest forms of physical activity are those that can be incorporated into everyday life.

Often when I talk to people about fitness they immediately think of Olympic athletes or professional football players. Don't think in terms of fitness being that level of performance required for sport; 'sports fitness' is very specific to sport performance. Fitness for improving health and well-being gives you the ability to work, rest and play without undue fatigue and have enough energy in reserve for emergencies. In other words, fitness for health and well-being means being able to participate in regular, moderate-intensity physical activity that can be maintained throughout your life. By implication, you can expect a better quality of life and a longer life.

Improving fitness for health and well-being needs to focus on the following four components:

- Flexibility of muscles and joints
- Muscular strength
- Muscular endurance
- Cardiovascular endurance

Exercise, unlike most other interventions such as dieting and medication, has the potential to benefit all elements of well-being (physical, psychological, social and spiritual). The benefits of exercise are far more than the visible, outward signs: improved mental health, lowered cholesterol and blood pressure and a reduced risk of chronic disease are additional significant gains in overall well-being.

A sobering statistic appeared in one World Health Organisation report in 2002: physical inactivity is one of the ten leading causes of death in developed countries, accounting for 1.9 million deaths per year worldwide. That is a needless loss of human life. My aim with this book is to provide you with ways to increase your levels of physical activity to achieve the recommended 150 minutes of exercise per week by making it part of your daily routine, creating opportunities for exercise wherever you are or whatever you are doing, and making it interesting, challenging, progressive and – most important – enjoyable.

1

Why should I bother exercising?

Physical activity levels have fallen dramatically in recent times despite the well-recognised health benefits of exercise and improved fitness. Many factors of modern life have contributed to the progressive reduction in physical activity: fewer manual jobs, less physically demanding housework and other chores such as shopping, a greater reliance on cars even for short distances, a lack of recreational facilities, and the high cost of accessing those facilities. In addition, our busy lifestyles make finding time for exercise more and more difficult. Indeed, the reason most people give for not exercising is lack of time.

How much exercise?

Most of us understand and accept that exercise is good for our health and well-being but the question is how much? The current physical activity guidelines of five 30-minute episodes a week of moderate-intensity physical activity equate to an energy expenditure of about 500–1,000 calories (equivalent to walking 6–12 miles per week). This level of physical activity reduces the risk of early death by 20–30 per cent. Furthermore, physically active individuals report a higher quality of life. The more exercise you do, the lower your risk of disease. In other words, exercise will add years to your life as well as life to your years! The message is: 'something is better than nothing;' do what exercise you can and attempt to increase it over weeks and months to reach the recommended 150 minutes a week. In my coaching experience, gradually increasing the amount of time you spend exercising is far more successful than an instant and dramatic increase in your exercise programme.

Even with elite athletes I introduce small but steady changes to their volume of training. Adopting a 'New Year's resolution mentality' to exercise, going from inactivity to athlete overnight, has the same success rate as dieting – it works for a month! It is incredible what you can achieve in a short space of time when you gradually increase exercise. And because a gradual increase is more manageable it becomes integral to your life, which means you are much more likely to maintain your exercise programme in the long term. Quite simply, it works. Swimming ace David Walliams could just about manage a mile when I first started coaching him but by small increases in his programme he was able to swim over 25 miles just 33 weeks later!

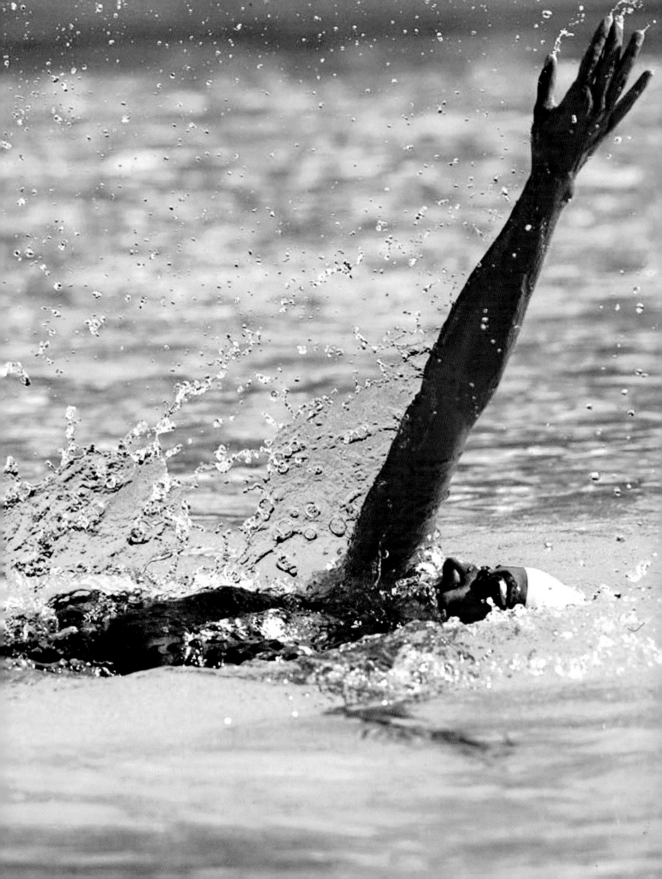

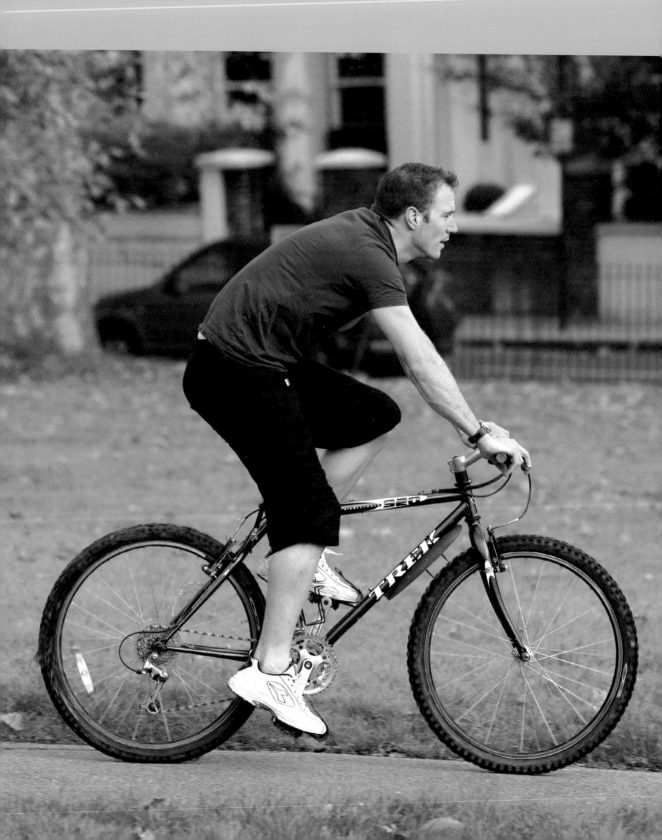

There is growing evidence in support of spreading out shorter bouts of physical activity over the day. For example, to make it easier to fit the recommended daily 30 minutes of moderate-intensity physical activity into your busy routine you can split it up, say into six 5-minute bouts throughout the day or four 5-minute bouts plus one 10-minute bout. By using this idea of 'portions' of exercise you are much more likely to achieve your overall 'exercise diet' of 150 minutes per week.

At your pace

The most demoralising aspect of exercise is when it is too hard. Exercise does not have to be vigorous (high intensity) to improve our fitness and health. The commonest reason I see for people failing to maintain an exercise programme is that it is so hard it becomes unenjoyable. You should always enjoy exercise and, while it may be a slog sometimes, overall it should be fun and make you want to come back for more.

When I coached four girls (Lynn, Mel, Pat and Sally) to swim the English Channel for the TV programme *This Morning* we all knew it was going to be very difficult, and at times downright miserable! Good things don't come easy and you just have to accept that some sessions will be hard work. It really helps to plan your exercise to optimise motivation and maintain your routine in the long term.

Setting goals (see Chapter 4) is an important way of motivating yourself. I used lots of different ways to motivate Lynn, Mel, Pat and Sally to achieve what most people felt was impossible. One of the motivational tools I used was focusing 'my' girls on how impressed people who were important to them would be with their achievement. At other times I would help them realise that

the enormity of the challenge would change their lives for the better and would redefine them as strong characters with their own identity. Each girl had her own motivating reason for taking part in the challenge and her own psychological and physiological barriers to overcome. Tapping into what would work for them as individuals was key. Mel, for example, was petrified of deep, open water – a real problem for a Channel swimmer! In addition, being part of a team was another important part of the girls' success; supporting one another through the good and bad times was crucial. The goal of swimming across the English Channel is a big motivator in itself, however, although such a significant challenge was also daunting. To overcome this I set the girls smaller goals along the way, such as swimming in open water for an hour, swimming solo for 3½ miles, and swimming from the mainland to the Isle of Wight. Using short- and long-term goals can be all the motivation you need – you don't have to be attempting the Channel!

Fitness: a friend for life

Good health is tied in with physical, mental, social and spiritual well-being; it's not solely the absence of disease. So why make so much of exercise? Well, it's because physical activity goes far beyond weight management. Physical activity is such a fundamental human behaviour that it is able to influence most major body systems, including our circulation, digestion and respiration. Increased levels of physical activity and fitness are directly linked to a reduction in the development of over 20 chronic diseases (for example, heart disease, diabetes and cancer). There is a number of important psychological benefits too, such as improved mood, reduced anxiety and boosted self-confidence. Furthermore, exercise can improve your social life simply by giving you opportunities to meet new people.

Added to these direct benefits, exercise indirectly leads to a healthier lifestyle by raising your chances of successfully dieting or giving up smoking. In part these positive outcomes reflect higher self-esteem and self-confidence and greater awareness of the advantages of healthy living. Research shows that making changes that accommodate regular exercise means that you are more likely to maintain a healthy lifestyle, a result that dieting or trying to stop smoking alone rarely achieves. It is a sad fact that only 10 per cent of those who diet are able to maintain weight loss in the long term.

Coronary heart disease and strokes

Cardiovascular disease is the most prevalent cause of death and reduced quality of life in the UK, resulting in over 200,000 deaths per year (40 per cent of all deaths). While a number of factors cause cardiovascular disease, it is indisputable that people who are physically active have a reduced risk of suffering heart disease or strokes. Higher levels of fitness can lessen the negative effects of other risk factors including smoking, high cholesterol levels and high blood pressure. People with diabetes, who are at a higher risk of developing cardiovascular disease, appear to benefit more from increased physical activity – even a small amount can reduce the risk of coronary heart disease. Exercise does not need to be vigorous to protect against cardiovascular disease but shorter, higher-intensity sessions can have the same positive effect as longer, lower-intensity sessions if the amount of energy expended is the same. Ten minutes of higher-intensity exercise can be as valuable as 30 minutes at a lower intensity, so you can accumulate the positive effects with smaller portions of exercise from 5 minutes upwards.

Hypertension (high blood pressure)

Exercise can be a potent ally in preventing and treating high blood pressure. All forms of exercise (strength and aerobic) are valuable in controlling high blood pressure. Physical activity works directly on the mechanisms responsible for controlling your blood pressure, thereby improving your body's ability to reduce the risk of hypertension, and indirectly by reducing your weight and lowering insulin resistance.

Diabetes

Diabetes affects the body's ability to store glucose. Two types of the disease are recognised. Type 1 diabetes occurs early in life and is associated with an inability to produce insulin, the hormone that controls the concentration of glucose in the blood. Type 2, which develops in later life, is associated with an inability to absorb and store glucose. Physical inactivity is a major risk factor for the development of Type 2 diabetes. People who are physically active have up to a 50 per cent lower risk of developing Type 2 diabetes and exercise can be effective even without weight loss. In other words, simply increasing your physical activity levels will do the job!

Physical inactivity and low fitness carries the same risk of heart disease as being a regular smoker!

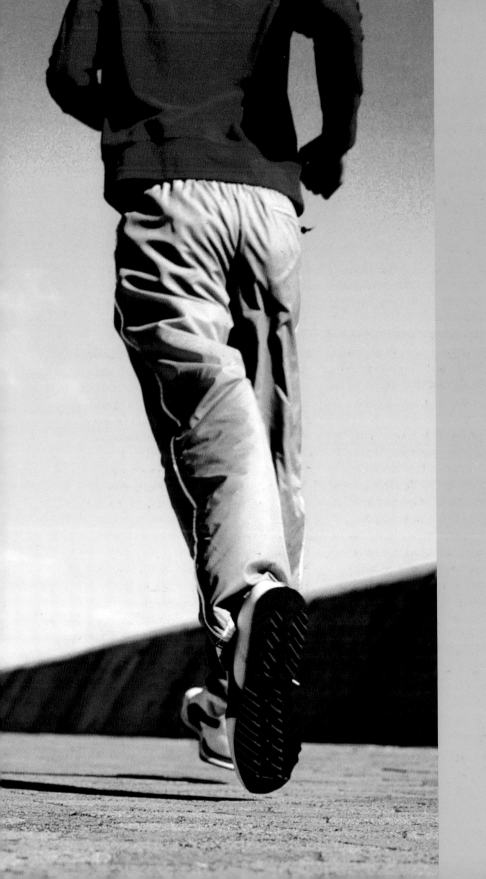

Prevention is better than cure! Increasing your physical activity levels before you develop abnormal glucose levels can be more effective in preventing Type 2 diabetes

For those with Type 2 diabetes it can improve blood glucose control. As with other chronic diseases, any exercise is beneficial, with the best results associated with programmes that combine strength and endurance exercise. Hard- or high-intensity exercise appears to be more effective in controlling diabetes than either medium- or low-intensity exercise.

Cancer

Cancer is the second largest cause of premature death in the UK, accounting for over 120,000 deaths per year. A large number of cancers are associated with a variety of lifestyle factors including diet, smoking, alcohol and inactivity. All types of exercise can help to reduce the chances of developing cancer, particularly the risk of colon, breast, lung and endometrial cancer, with moderate- or high-intensity exercise proving to be the most effective.

Osteoporosis (brittle bone disease)

People suffering from osteoporosis have an increased risk of bone fracture. This degenerative bone disease results in low bone mass and strength. During adolescence we are able to increase our bone mass, but in middle and later life we need to exercise to maintain bone mineral density to offset the inevitable reduction in bone mass. For bone health, we need to focus on activities

that produce high physical stresses on the bone, such as running, jumping and skipping. Strength exercises are also beneficial as they increase the loading stress on the bones.

Musculo-skeletal health (low back pain and osteoarthritis)

Over 80 per cent of people in the UK suffer back pain at some time during their lives. Back pain is bad news for the economy (one report found that as many as 150 million work days per year were lost through back trouble), and for the individual the most profound problem is reduced quality of life. Aerobic-type exercise (see Chapter 6) helps to prevent back pain and reduce the chance of it being a recurring problem. The type of exercise is not important, although I would not recommend prolonged exercise because fatigue may increase the possibility of injury. In addition to aerobic activity, exercises to improve core stability and strength endurance (see pages 44–71 and 163) of abdominal and back muscles are beneficial in reducing the incidence of low back pain. As well as improving your functional capacity, exercise for low back pain has psychological benefits, including greater confidence and self-esteem.

The commonest disorder of the joints in middle-aged and older people is osteoarthritis which affects the hands, hips, shoulders and knees. It is the most frequently occurring form of arthritis and is a major cause of a reduced quality of life and disability. With this condition the cartilage that protects the ends of the bones breaks down, causing pain and swelling. Even though joint pain is often increased when the affected joint is used, maintaining activity is important to protect the joint, reduce pain and remain mobile. Several factors can accelerate the development of osteoarthritis, among them trauma injury to the joint surface, obesity and inactivity. Obesity appears to cause metabolic changes in the cartilage and an increase in weight puts pressure on the joint and can result in permanent damage. By contrast, inactivity fails to exert adequate mechanical forces on our cartilage to promote its growth and repair. It is therefore vital to continue to be physically active, particularly in later life, to optimise the growth and repair of joint cartilage, maintain a healthy weight and protect our joints. All types of exercise are effective in reducing pain, stiffness and disability.

Mental health

Depression is a growing problem in the UK and elsewhere. Physical activity significantly aids our mental health by improving mood and reducing stress and anxiety levels. This gain in physical self-perception and self-esteem is important in reducing the development of mental illness. All forms of exercise can help to prevent or treat mental illness and enhance our mental health. And since the effects of exercise are different for each of us, tailoring your programme to optimise your enjoyment makes exercise more effective.

There are physiological and psychological reasons why exercise leads to that 'feel-good factor'. Physiological factors include the release in the body of chemicals (called endorphins) that lead to a feeling of improved well-being. The release of these naturally occurring opiate-like substances results in what we commonly call 'runner's high'. Other chemicals, including dopamine and serotonin, which are involved in nerve transport in the brain, are released in greater quantities during exercise and this causes the 'buzz' we often experience afterwards. It has been suggested that simply increasing body temperature through exercise reduces anxiety, in a similar way as taking a hot bath or a sauna does. In psychological terms, it may be that exercise simply distracts you from the stresses of daily life that create anxiety. Relaxation can have a similar effect, although the impact of exercise lasts longer than relaxation alone. Another psychological factor that improves mental health is the concept of 'mastery'. When you start a new exercise there is a real sense of achievement and self-satisfaction when you begin to master it. New exercises also make fitness sessions more interesting and the net result is that you are more likely to maintain your new exercise regime.

Another important component in mental health is sleep. Unfortunately, a third of adults in the UK report sleep problems. Exercise is closely linked with improved sleep quality. Physically active individuals fall asleep faster, and sleep longer and more deeply than inactive individuals.

So, why should we bother exercising? Because quite simply it is the easiest, cheapest and most effective way to improve your chances of a long, happy and healthy life.

Mental illness in the form of depression is set to become the second most prevalent cause of disability worldwide by 2020. Physical activity is effective in preventing and treating mental illness and is as effective as psychotherapy and medication.

2

Surely I can diet and save myself the energy?

Obesity is a growing problem throughout the Western world. In the UK almost a quarter of men and women are classed as clinically obese and the number of severely overweight children and adolescents is a major cause for concern. Obesity is associated with excessive weight and is measured in a number of different ways. The most commonly used method is the body mass index (BMI), expressed as: body weight (kg) divided by height squared (m²). Although it seems simple enough, this and other commonly used methods fail to assess body composition, in other words what percentage of body weight is muscle rather than fat. Distinguishing between fat mass and non-fat mass is important in identifying the potential risks of excessive weight (muscle mass is beneficial for health whereas excessive fat is detrimental). Highly muscular individuals (strength-trained athletes, for instance) often have a very high BMI but this may not be linked with an increased risk of disease.

When you start a new exercise programme it's important to understand body composition. If you use body weight as your measure of success, do be aware that muscle weighs more than fat and an increase

in muscle mass while lowering your fat mass can result in no overall weight loss – or even in weight gain. Therefore, you should not feel downhearted at not having lost any weight because the reality is that you have made positive changes to your body composition, leading to improved health and well-being. Since there are no easy ways to assess body composition, rather than using weight-related goals, I'd encourage you to think about using other targets.

What causes obesity?

Obesity is the visible indication of an individual in positive energy balance. In other words, obesity is a sign of inactivity and excessive calorie consumption. Weight management is very easy to understand: if you eat more calories than you burn you will put weight on (a 'positive energy balance'), if you eat fewer calories than you burn you will lose weight (a 'negative energy balance') and if you eat and burn up the same number of calories you will maintain your weight ('energy balance') – see page 20. The amount of energy we burn is a combination of our 'resting metabolic rate' (the amount of energy we burn at rest to support normal function) plus the amount

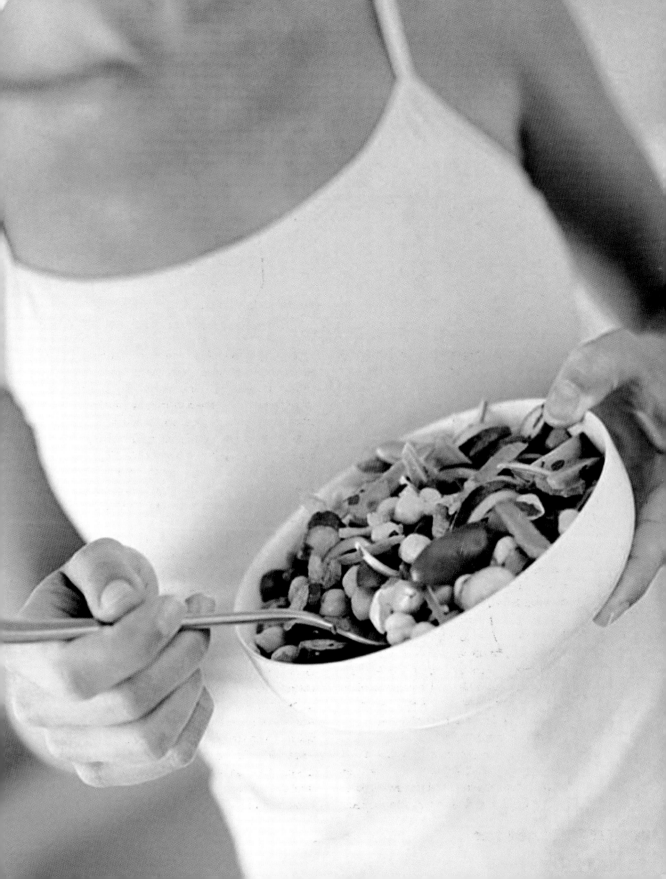

The energy balance

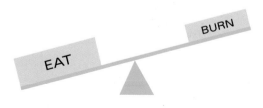

Weight gain
Positive energy balance – when the number of calories eaten is greater than the number of calories burnt

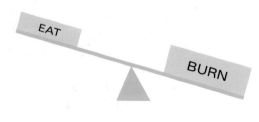

Weight loss
Negative energy balance – when the number of calories eaten is less than the number of calories burnt

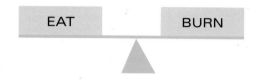

Weight maintenance
Energy balance – when the number of calories eaten is equal to the number of calories burnt

of calories we burn during physical activity (ranging from housework to exercise). So it is really very simple: to lose weight we can either reduce the number of calories we eat (diet), increase the number of calories we burn (exercise) or both. The most successful weight-management programmes are the combined result of eating less and increasing physical activity.

Why hasn't the diet message worked?
Despite a tidal wave of information and education about diet, obesity persists as a major health problem in the West. The number of overweight and obese individuals continues to rise. The UK is a fatter nation than it was just 20 years ago. Evidence suggests that even though we have managed to lower the average number of calories we consume, we are still getting fatter. The reason is simply that we are becoming progressively less active (remember the energy balance), so although we are eating fewer calories we are also burning less energy. Unfortunately, the reduction in physical activity is greater than the reduction in the number of calories we eat. Driven by a multi-million-pound diet industry and a media obsessed with diet, we continue to reinforce the message that dieting is the only way to control weight. Yes, diet is an important weapon in the fight against obesity, but on its own eating less is relatively impotent without an increase in physical activity.

Size 0 and eating disorders
Our obsession with weight loss through diet alone is resulting in health issues that are equally as problematic as those associated with obesity in some individuals. The media

focus is on dieting to lose weight, recently through the example of size 0 models. Closer inspection of their lifestyles shows that they use both diet and exercise to control their weight. Models rarely talk about exercise yet the vast majority have personal trainers! People who strive to make their bodies ultra-thin are led to believe that dieting is the only way to lose weight. Many make themselves unhappy and ill by severely restricting their calorific intake. Eating disorders, including bulimia and anorexia nervosa, are on the increase in the UK, particularly among women. These disorders must be addressed quickly, usually with help from a psychiatrist, before associated health problems set in, such as diseases associated with malnutrition and either disruption or loss of the menstrual cycle that may negatively impact on bone mineral density and fertility levels.

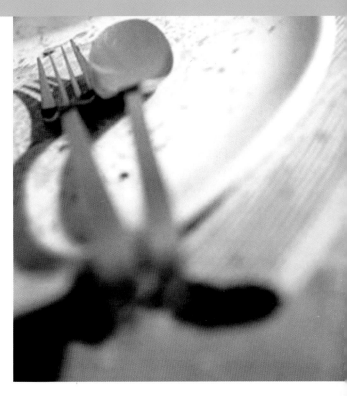

What is the most effective way to manage weight?

The best way to lose weight and keep it off is by a combination of physical activity (exercise) and calorific restriction (diet). This approach maximises weight loss in the form of fat mass while helping to maintain muscle mass. Maintaining your muscle mass is important as this is where the vast majority of calories are burned. Dieting without exercising leads to a loss of muscle mass and in turn reduces the number of calories you burn at rest, decreasing your resting metabolic rate. As a consequence you will need further to reduce the number of calories you eat to maintain the same amount of weight loss. It's a downward spiral that continues until your calorific intake is so low that you run significant health risks. It is far better to combine a well-balanced, healthy diet with increased levels of physical activity. This dual approach offers the safest and most effective strategy for weight management.

All forms of exercise are beneficial for weight management. As well as increasing the number of calories you burn, strength exercises improve your ability to carry out the tasks of daily life and you'll feel less tired. We know that exercise is also effective in reducing the development of chronic disease and improving mental health. It makes you feel good and improves your social life too. Even if exercise seems like a chore initially, there are lots of ways to enhance the experience and once it is part of your life you will really look forward to it. Compare that to dieting alone, which is never enjoyable, rarely improves your mood, often increases your anxiety and has no positive impact on your social life!

3

How do I structure my workouts?

To maximise the benefits of exercise in the short and long term there is a number of key principles that you should use to plan and structure your workouts. Even after two decades in the industry, when I am designing an exercise programme I always return to these principles. Adhering to these rules will help you understand the benefits you gain from different types of exercise and will make it easy to design an exercise programme that targets the areas of fitness that are important to you.

I always begin with the goals of the person in order to identify their immediate and future targets and construct a programme that will really work for them. I also establish their physical condition and exercise experience, and the type of exercise they enjoy, before starting to design the programme. Armed with this information I use a set of principles of structuring exercise to design a bespoke programme that offers the greatest opportunity for success: progressive overload, volume (intensity, frequency and duration), reversibility, specificity and individuality, and recovery. Adhering to these principles ensures a safe and effective programme that can be maintained in the long term.

Equilibrium

The body remains in a balanced state (called 'equilibrium' or 'homeostasis') until it is acted upon by something that stresses the body's systems. Stressors include environmental factors such as heat and cold, stressful situations and exercise. In trying to maintain equilibrium the body responds to stressors in several ways. For example, in response to heat the body redirects blood to the skin, causing the familiar red flushing of the skin, and begins to sweat in an attempt to remove heat from the body and regulate body temperature.

Exercise is a potent stressor that affects all systems in the body. A single bout of exercise can result in a wide range of acute responses, including an increase in energy consumption, heart rate, breathing volume, oxygen consumption, carbon dioxide production, blood pressure and body temperature. These are the body's attempt to maintain equilibrium. Once you stop exercising the responses subside: heart and breathing rates rapidly fall, body temperature slowly falls and energy consumption begins to return to resting levels. The harder the exercise and the longer its duration, the longer it takes for the body's systems to return to resting levels.

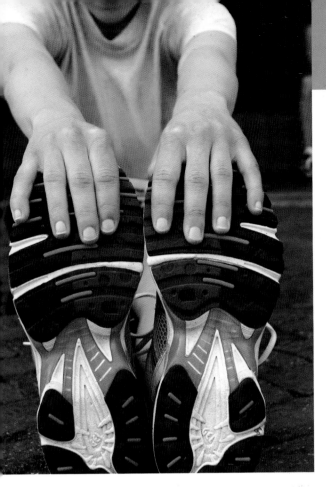

If a form of stress is placed on the body repetitively over a prolonged period of time, the acute responses observed following a single bout of exercise lead to adaptation of the body's systems in order to achieve a new balance point. As a result of this resetting of equilibrium the body is better able to cope with the stress on it. Because all of the body's systems – cardiovascular, pulmonary, skeletal, hormonal – respond to acute bouts of stress, they can all adapt to the stress to regain equilibrium. What this means in terms of your health and fitness is that you will see a net improvement in your systems' capability in response to repeated bouts of exercise over time: your muscles are stronger, your joints more flexible, your heart and lungs more efficient, and you feel more mentally alert.

Exercise is, of course, a positive stimulus, but unfortunately there are also negative ones to which our body's systems have to adapt (or rather maladapt): inactivity, poor diet, smoking, and forms of emotional and mental stress. The key is to reduce the negative stimuli and increase the positive adaptations.

Progressive overload

For adaptation to take place the body's systems require a stimulus greater than the system has previously encountered: this is termed 'overload'. With respect to fitness, the adaptive process requires a sufficient volume of exercise (that is, of sufficient intensity, duration and frequency – see pages 24–26) to ensure an overload and resultant adaptive response.

To continue to improve, the exercise overload must be progressive, constantly increasing the stimulus to bring about adaptation. This process is termed 'progressive overload' and is a critical component in designing an exercise programme to ensure that you continue to adapt (improve) in the long term. Progressive overload is also important when setting goals and in motivating you to continue your exercise programme in the long term.

In my experience, progressive overload is often the key factor in designing a successful programme. I always build flexibility into a programme. Don't see it as set in stone – it should be always be possible to change it to suit you. If you feel you are progressing too quickly, slow the rate of progression rather than feel discouraged and give up. If you are fed up with your programme, change it. As anyone I have ever worked with will tell you, I continually monitor my programmes and make changes immediately if they are

Volume of exercise

Volume simply refers to how much exercise you complete in a set period of time (day, week, month or year). The volume of exercise has three components: intensity, duration and frequency. Intensity relates to how hard the exercise is for a given session, duration relates to how long you exercise in that session and frequency relates to how often you exercise.

training volume =
intensity x duration x frequency

In other words:

**how much =
how hard x how long x how often**

Increasing the volume of exercise is important in maintaining a progressive overload to ensure your continual improvement in the long term. Try to increase the volume of individual sessions as well as your weekly or monthly volume. Monitoring your training volume can be very complex but if you assign a point score to your sessions that will give you a session-by-session volume. The cumulative total of this session-by-session volume will give you exercise volume over a week, month or year. In the main section of this book exercise sessions are broken down into 5-, 10- and 30-minute portions and intensity is ranked easy, medium or hard.

Use the following ranking system to calculate exercise volume for a single session:

Duration

5 minutes = 5 points

10 minutes = 10 points

30 minutes = 30 points

Intensity

easy = 1 point

medium = 2 points

hard = 3 points

A 5-minute session at a hard intensity =
5 points x 3 points = **15 points**

A 5-minute session at a medium intensity =
5 points x 2 points = **10 points**

A 30-minute session at an easy intensity =
30 points x 1 point = **30 points**

A 30-minute walk at an easy intensity that includes three 5-minute periods at a medium intensity scores as follows:

15 minutes at an easy pace =
15 points x 1 point = **15 points**

Plus:
15 minutes at a medium pace =
15 points x 2 points = **30 points**

Session volume total of:
15 points + 30 points = **45 points**

I often use this approach to monitor training volume for several reasons:

• It's easy to understand and keep track of weekly and monthly exercise volume by adding up individual training-session volumes.

• The ease of tracking progression means it's ideal for setting short-term goals, such as achieving a certain number of points in a week.

• It's possible to identify problem times: if an individual is constantly picking up injuries or illness I can look at the volume and see if the two are related.

• It allows changes in exercise volume to be made quickly and easily.

Intensity This is related to how hard you are working and is a measure of how much energy an activity demands. In general, the amount of energy required for a given exercise is the same for individuals of similar weight. The larger you are, the more energy is required for a given exercise. (This applies only for exercises that require you to carry your weight.) As your fitness increases, the intensity of the same exercise falls: that is, it gets easier. To continue improving you must continually increase the difficulty of the exercise so that you are overloading the system (progressive overload). There is a number of ways to achieve an overload: for 30-minute and 10-minute exercises maintaining the target intensity (easy, medium or hard) will ensure you are always achieving an overload because as you get fitter you will be able to do more exercise – for example, walk further for the same intensity.

In general, I find intensity to be the most potent way of changing exercise volume, though I am always careful when increasing intensity as even small increases can rapidly lead to excessive fatigue, injury and illness. I increase the intensity only by a small amount and in a small number of exercise bouts at any one time. On the plus side, because intensity is such a potent stimulus to exercise volume you can increase training volume without increasing the number of sessions or duration of sessions. The net result is an improvement in your fitness that doesn't take up more of your free time! Chapter 7 gives you ways of monitoring the intensity of exercise, including psychological and physiological responses to exercise.

Duration This is simply how long you exercise in each session. Often the duration of exercise is dictated by the intensity; hard exercise (high intensity) can be maintained only for short bouts while easy exercise (low intensity) can be sustained for prolonged periods. Increasing the duration of exercise is an effective way of maintaining the required stimulus to achieve overload without having to increase intensity. Increasing duration rather than intensity can often be an easier way of increasing volume as your perception of effort is the same except that you are exercising for longer.

Frequency This refers to the number of times you exercise in a set period. Usually I use a day or a week as the period of time although longer periods can be adopted when planning long-term goals. Increasing the frequency of exercise (how many times in a set period) will also maintain the required stimulus to achieve overload. It should be your goal to exercise on as many days of the week as possible, however; take every opportunity to exercise and don't worry if you find it difficult to fit in exercise on a particular day, you can always increase the number of sessions on other days in the week.

Reversibility

Exercise is not a short-term fix. The benefits of exercise are lost once you stop exercising, a principle termed reversibility or regression. Try to think about exercise as a positive lifestyle change, an integral part of everyday life rather than an add-on. To help you do this, your programme should be tailored for your specific needs and lifestyle. If you focus on what is important to you and set yourself goals that you wish to achieve, that will motivate you to strive for them. If you are able

to maintain exercise continually it becomes easier and more enjoyable. Exercising for only short, concentrated periods at certain times of the year (because it was your New Year's resolution, because you want to look good on the beach in the summer, or just to look your best for special occasions) can be really hard work because all the adaptations you gained from your previous exercise programme have been lost with inactivity. Through reversibility your fitness level will have dropped and you have to start at the beginning again – the hardest part of any exercise programme.

I often advise people simply to change their exercise programme rather than stop exercise completely. Switching to a completely new exercise or joining up with a 'buddy' (see page 35) can be enough to maintain your physical activity. Team games such as basketball or 5-a-side football are one way to add variety to a programme. And variety is the spice of a successful exercise programme! By exercising on a regular basis you maintain the adaptations made by your body's systems and that way certain events in the year become the motivation to increase your exercise volume from your existing programme. The more you do, the less effort is required, and you will maximise the health benefits in the short and long term.

Specificity and individuality

Specificity refers to adaptations to exercise that are directly associated with the type of exercise you undertake. It is linked to the energy systems (aerobic, speed, power), muscle groups (legs, arms and so on) and skill (movements that closely mimic those of the target skill, such as skiing) used in specific exercises. For example, strength exercises improve strength in certain muscles that an

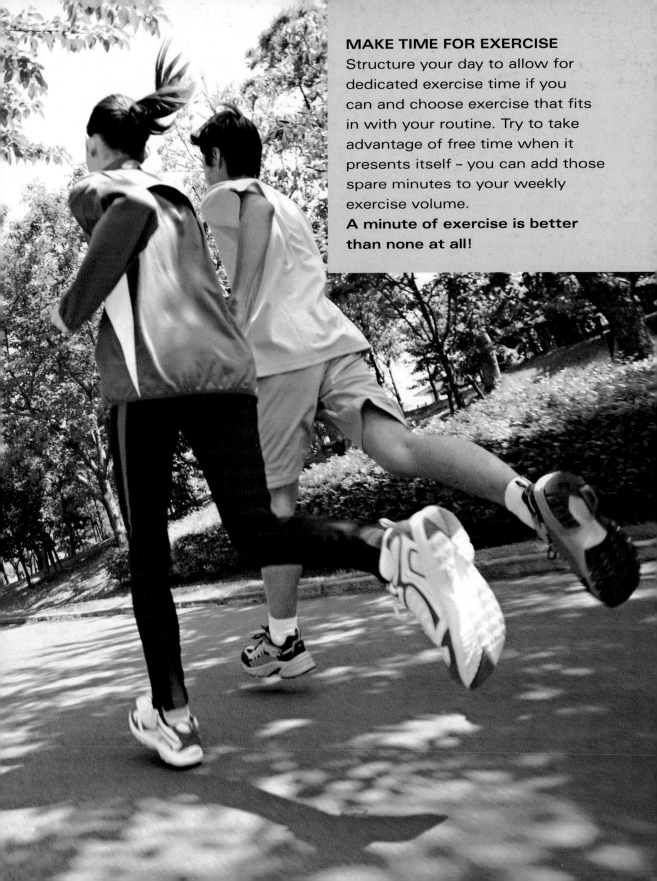

MAKE TIME FOR EXERCISE
Structure your day to allow for dedicated exercise time if you can and choose exercise that fits in with your routine. Try to take advantage of free time when it presents itself – you can add those spare minutes to your weekly exercise volume.

A minute of exercise is better than none at all!

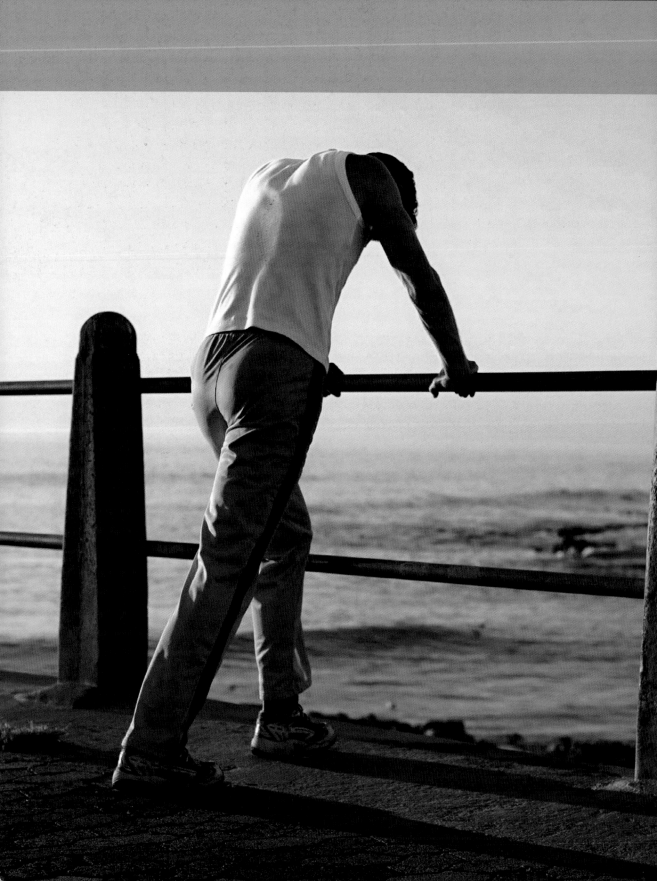

exercise focuses on, such as squats (see page 92), which improve leg strength without a gain in upper body strength; medium-intensity aerobic exercise, say walking or jogging, improves aerobic capacity (your ability to use oxygen); and 5- and 10-minute exercises at a hard intensity improve anaerobic capacity (your speed and strength endurance). (The word stamina is often used to describe aerobic or cardiovascular endurance. Strength endurance is also termed muscular endurance.)

To optimise the benefits of exercise, choose exercises that focus specifically on the components of fitness and those muscle groups that will allow you to achieve your goal. If the aim is to reduce lower back pain you should select exercises that improve the strength of the core muscles (stomach and back) and the strength endurance of those muscle groups. Easy- and medium-intensity exercise also reduces low back pain and should therefore be part of your exercise programme. Selecting exercises that are specific to your goals will gain you the greatest adaptation in the fastest time.

We are all individuals: our goals are different and we respond differently to types of exercise. Some people adapt very rapidly to stresses and require a limited amount of recovery. Others adapt very slowly and require longer periods of recovery to optimise the adaptive process. Think carefully about the volume of exercise and how much recovery time is appropriate to you and your needs. Don't be surprised if your exercise programme is unlike that of your friends. Tailoring a programme that targets your specific needs is essential, which is why it's worth considering a session with a personal trainer. See Chapter 8 for training programmes.

Sleep is an important part of the regenerative process too, Research suggests that recovery from exercise is greatest during sleep. In addition, obesity is more prevalent in those who sleep the least. Enjoy that sleep: it's good for you!

Recovery

Making sure you give your body time to recover is crucial in optimising adaptation to exercise. Placing an overload on the body results in fatigue and you need to allow a period of rest and recovery to enable the body to adapt, to the exercise stimulus. Without recovery the body does not have time to adapt and unless you plan enough recovery into your programme you will be in a constant state of fatigue without any real improvement in fitness. That said, if you allow too much recovery you lose the adaptations that you have gained – remember reversibility!

Plan recovery in your exercise programme and think about having a day without exercise in the week. This will ensure your body can adapt and you have a day off to recharge your batteries and prepare for the following week's exercise. I always suggest the recovery day can be flexible; rather than prescribing a set day you can fit a rest day around work or family commitments or simply take it when you can't be bothered or are too tired. I also leave a variable number of days between rest days: say, 3 days' exercise, 1 day's rest, 4 days' exercise, 1 day's rest. This adds variety as the rest day changes every week and there are never more than 4 consecutive days of exercise.

Plan and structure your exercise

The most successful exercise programmes are those that are planned and well structured. Planning exercise into dedicated times of the week helps to ensure you don't miss sessions and assists in maintaining your exercise in the long term. Exercising with someone else makes a big difference: it's far more difficult to miss a session that you have planned with a friend.

Structure your exercise to fit in with your daily life. Using periods of the day when you have no other commitments or times when you would normally be sitting around doing nothing constructive makes motivating yourself to exercise much easier. That said,

don't be too rigid with your plan – seize the chance to exercise if it arises. If you find yourself watching rubbish on TV take the opportunity to squeeze in 5, 10 or 30 minutes of exercise. A well-planned and structured exercise programme should be effortless to achieve.

Starting exercise for the first time

To avoid injury and soreness, start off with a small amount of easy exercise and gradually build up the volume (intensity, duration and frequency) over time. Monitor your exercise volume to ensure that you are progressing at a rate that suits you. Avoid massive increases in exercise volume in short periods of time. Even

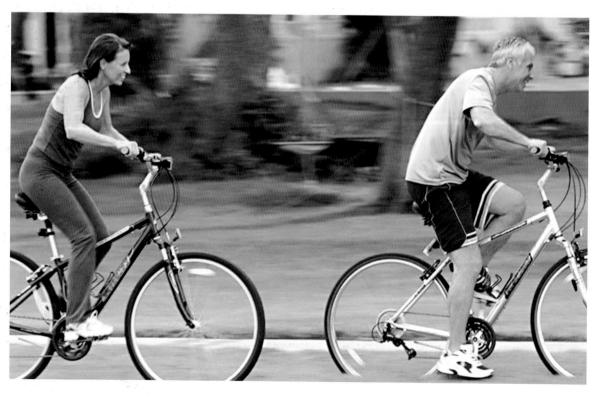

for the experienced exerciser a rapid increase in volume can lead to injury and illness.

Because exercise does place extra stress upon the body's systems, be aware there are some risks for individuals with an existing disease, and it is not always obvious if you have a disease that may be affected by exercise. Answering the questions in the panel on the right will give you some idea of whether you have a condition that may be affected by exercise. If you answer yes to any of these, consult your GP before starting your exercise programme. If you have a diagnosed chronic health problem – heart disease, lung disease or diabetes, or are at a high risk of developing any these diseases – again consult your GP before starting exercise.

It is important to remember that exercise is beneficial in preventing and treating chronic disease. Even if you have been diagnosed with a disease, exercise is rarely discouraged – rather, the opposite: exercise is often encouraged more vigorously for anyone with a chronic disease. The one difference is that the approach is somewhat more cautious, starting exercise at easy intensities and progressing at a slower rate than those without disease. Unfortunately, in my experience, it is people with chronic disease who feel less able to exercise or who are more afraid of the possible problems if they do. I have designed exercise programmes for some of the most vulnerable patients and understand these concerns. Such individuals often have the most to gain from exercise and I suggest that a cautious approach, in close consultation with the medical community and a personal trainer, will help allay fears and promote an active lifestyle. I give the same advice to anyone starting exercise for the first time or returning to exercise after a long period of inactivity.

Questions to ask before you exercise for the first time

Before you start exercising for the first time or restart exercise, having stopped for a long period, answer the following questions:

Has your doctor ever told you that you have a heart condition?

Do you feel pain in your chest during physical activity?

Have you recently suffered from chest pain at rest?

Do you suffer from dizziness?

Have you ever lost consciousness?

Do you suffer from joint problems that may be made worse by exercise?

Are you currently taking drugs for high blood pressure, high cholesterol or a heart condition?

Do you know of any other reason why you should not participate in exercise?

If you have answered yes to any of the questions or if you are over the age of 40 years and are inactive, consult your GP before you start exercising. If you answered no to all of these questions, it is likely that you can safely start to exercise.

4

How can I motivate myself to exercise?

Humans are programmed to exercise; it's part of our make-up. As babies we are motivated to exercise: first to kick, then to crawl and then walk; we learn how to hit balls and do so without encouragement or reward. As people get older, their motivation to exercise diminishes. The key to maximising the health and well-being benefits of physical activity is to make exercise an integral part of everyday life. And the way to do that is to develop an exercise programme that requires very little effort or motivation. I know that summoning the motivation to take up exercise in the first place and then pushing yourself to continue exercising in the long term can be very difficult, particularly for a first-time exerciser. Moving from very little or no exercise to clocking up 150 minutes per week can seem a daunting and unachievable task. Don't be put off! I have a number of ways of enhancing your motivation and improving the quality and longevity of exercise.

Setting goals

As someone once said to me: remember that you don't have to eat the elephant in one bite! Most of us are better at tackling something in smaller 'bites', or stages, and this is how

to go about fitting exercise into your life. By meeting short-term goals you build up to achieving your long-term goal (the whole elephant!). One of the best ways to motivate yourself is to have a target to aim for. Clearly identify your goal at the start of your exercise programme – it will give a real boost to your strategy. The goal itself can vary: you may want to lose weight, get fitter, reduce lower back pain, improve your upper body strength or just increase your physical activity levels. One goal that is always worth including is that you should strive to feel that you are good at exercising, and that you enjoy it. If you feel good about what you do, losing weight, getting fitter or gaining strength become a bonus to doing something you enjoy. Trying to find enjoyment in everything you do is a skill that should help in numerous aspects of life.

When setting out what you want to achieve, I think it helps to identify both short-term goals (ones to be met in, say, a week or a month) and long-term goals (those you want to be hitting in, say, 6 months to a year). Ensure the goals are achievable yet challenging; if you make them too easy you will get bored, but if they are too difficult you will lose interest, and either way you will

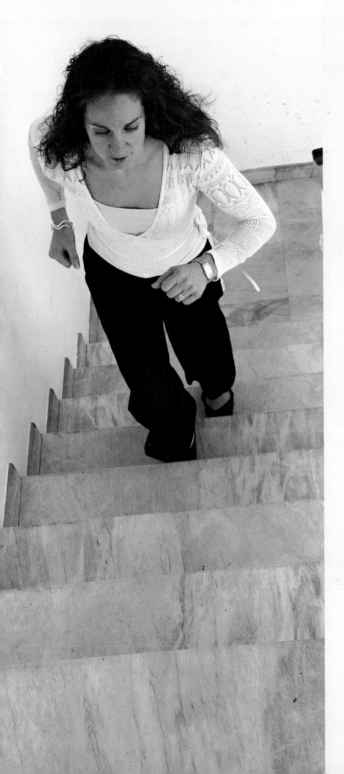

Setting successful goals

1 Set goals that are challenging but achievable: if a goal is too easy it won't motivate you. For your long-term goals, think about something you have always dreamed of achieving and believe you can do it: for example, the London–Brighton cycle ride or the London Marathon.

2 Use both short- and long-term goals. Include in your short-term goals setting a target for the number of lengths in one session or the number of sessions to complete in a week. Long-term goals might be a target body weight or running a long-distance race.

3 Build progression into your goals so that you continue to improve. For instance, you can progress by increasing the distance you walk in a week. If you cannot build in more time, progressively increase the intensity of each session instead.

4 Select exercises that fit into your lifestyle and that you are comfortable with. If you enjoy walking, set yourself walking goals. You need to be prepared for days when circumstances like bad weather prevent you going out, and have another stamina-building exercise lined up, such as stair climbing or swimming.

5 Reward yourself when you achieve your goal (but avoid using food as a reward!) and set the reward in line with the goal: big goal, big reward.

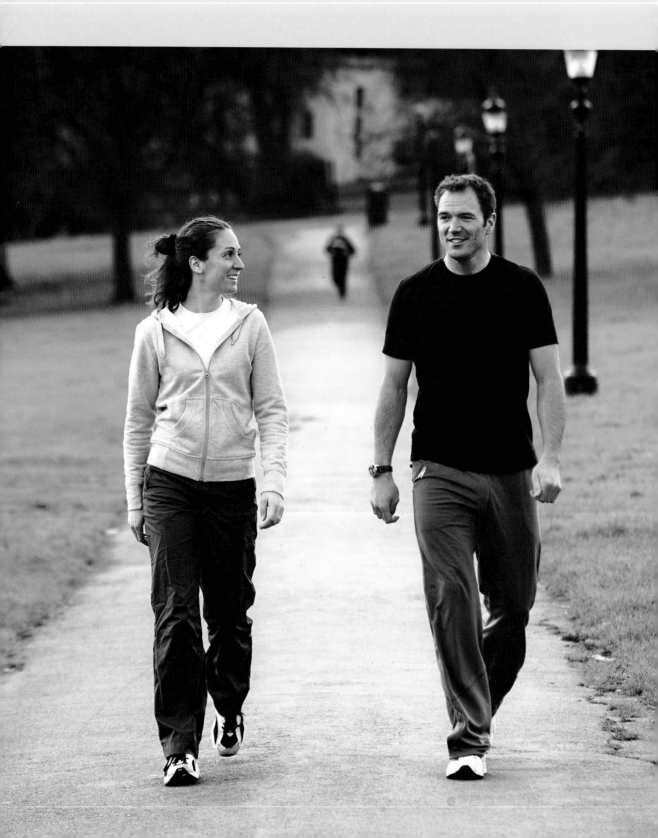

probably give up on your programme. Rather than looking at a physical outcome such as weight loss or increased strength (that may take some time to achieve), set goals that give results in the short term. For example, aim to increase the amount of time you spend exercising in a week – start at 15 minutes a week and increase by 5 minutes per week.

If you do use a physical outcome as your goal, think about making it a medium-term goal, over 3–6 months. Setting physical-outcome goals for periods shorter than this is rarely successful because it takes time for adaptation (see page 23) to take place. What tends to happen is that individuals become demotivated because they don't feel their progress has been quick enough.

Choose the right intensity

Getting the intensity of exercise right is crucial in the early stages of an exercise programme. Choosing to exercise at a high intensity is a common mistake for new exercisers and for those returning to exercise after a long period of inactivity. Inappropriately high exercise intensities can lead to severe fatigue, muscle soreness and possible injury. The outcome is a big drop-out rate during the early stages of an exercise programme despite motivation being relatively high. It is always better to start off easy and work up at a reasonable rate so that you develop a sense of progress. People get excited when they are moving quickly towards achieving their goals, which is why it is important to ensure that progress is being made. With this approach you will be able to monitor your progress and make adjustments to the intensity as necessary. Importantly, this strategy will dramatically enhance your enjoyment of exercise that will have a long-term impact.

Hard work doesn't have to be a misery. Exercise can be tough yet enjoyable. Adapt your exercise programme to ensure it is challenging but satisfying and create an environment that makes exercise more enjoyable.

Exercise with a friend

Exercising on your own can be a lonely experience. If you are exercising outdoors you may sometimes be reluctant to go out on your own for a whole variety of reasons. Having an 'exercise buddy' can increase your enjoyment of exercise and help you maintain your exercise programme. On days when you don't feel like exercising your 'buddy' will encourage you and vice versa, meaning that you are both much more likely to achieve your short- and long-term goals. It is important to discuss your goals with the your 'exercise buddy', emphasising that there will be times when motivation will wane, and that you will need to support each other to stick at it. You can also improve your chances of making a session by arranging to meet your 'buddy' at a certain time and place (the same time each week). That way you will have to attend the session to avoid letting your 'buddy' down.

Try to select the right 'exercise buddy' or group of people to exercise with, otherwise this strategy can be counter-productive. For example, consider the runner who joined a local running club with a view to improving motivation after a long break. After plucking up the courage to go, it can be highly demotivating if the existing runners are too fast. Struggling to keep up reinforces feelings

Motivational music to invigorate your session is often played loud for greatest effect. Soft music with a slow tempo can help relax you during low-intensity and stretching exercise.

of incompetence. Eventually the runner in this example gave up and never returned to the club. For the same reason, you need to team up with a person or people who don't make you feel you are not at their level. If the initial experience helps you feel good about your ability and about how you fit in, this too will build motivation.

Exercise with music

Music could play a major role in addressing the growing inactivity and obesity problem. Listening to music can really improve the quality of your workout, increase your overall enjoyment and help maintain your exercise programme in the long term. Research has shown that how you decide what music to listen to while exercising is closely linked to how that music is composed and performed, and how you interpret it. The way music has been put together – its composition and tempo and the instruments it is played on – can powerfully impact upon the listener. Some music is highly motivational for exercise just by its very nature: high-energy club anthems are great during hard sessions, as are rock and punk bands like U2 and the Clash. And of course certain pieces of music may mean something special to the listener and can have a highly motivational effect for this reason.

Music is particularly useful for low- or medium-intensity exercise. It can reduce your

perceived exertion (how hard you feel you're having to work), making this level of exercise feel easier, and in so doing can increase your enjoyment and help you maintain exercise long term. Music can be used to invigorate your session or to relax you, depending on your choice. For stretching exercises, soft music with a slow tempo can act as a sedative, reducing arousal levels, and can help you achieve a better range of motion and make you feel relaxed. In contrast, fast-tempo (say, over 120 beats per minute), invigorating music with a strong rhythm increases arousal and can enhance the positive aspects of mood such as vigour and happiness, while reducing the negative aspects including tension and possibly depression. This effect on our arousal levels is brought about because fast, upbeat music increases respiration rate, heart rate, sweat secretion and other indicators of physical activation. Arousal is also increased through music that promotes thoughts that inspire physical activity.

It's very easy to make your own compilation of music tracks that have a motivating effect for you and put them on a CD or MP3. It is worth emphasising that songs or music that motivate one person may not do the same for another. Two songs with the same beat can be interpreted very differently, for we all like different things. While this seems an obvious point, the important message is that you as an individual should spend some time selecting music that motivates you, regardless of whether or not it does the trick for anyone else. Use as many tracks as you can and try listening to them on 'shuffle' mode to avoid repeating the same music over and over again. Keeping the music updated and fresh will help maintain your motivation during exercise. You can even use

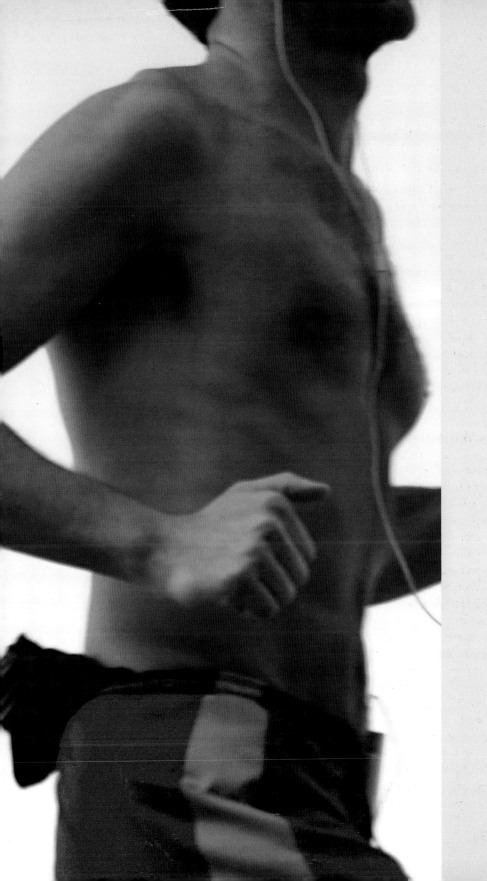

music before you exercise to motivate you – so if you are thinking you can't be bothered, try putting some music!

Reward yourself

Reward yourself when you reach your goals (short- and long-term). Give yourself something that you really want and let yourself have the reward only when you have truly earned it. Rewarding yourself will help develop your confidence in your ability to do exercise: people tend to enjoy activities that they are good at.

It is important that success is recognised and recorded. Allowing someone else to be the judge of whether you have achieved your goal removes any temptation to cheat and it adds value to the reward process by making it a prize-giving ceremony with public recognition of your achievement. Try to avoid using food or alcohol as a reward because achieving your exercise goals should not be linked to habits that are counter-productive to fitness. By making food, particularly calorie-dense foods such as cakes or chocolate, the reward you are reinforcing a subconscious message that you are punishing yourself by not having the reward. In other words, exercise becomes your punishment for eating snacks or treats.

Think inventively about the types of rewards you use for reaching your pre-determined target. For example, enjoy an extra hour in bed, or treat yourself to a manicure or a massage. Remember too that the size of reward should reflect the achievement and recognise the effort required to reach the goal. Attaining 90 minutes of exercise in a week merits that extra hour in bed, whereas buying yourself a new gadget or a massage should be your treat

for maintaining 150 minutes of exercise per week for 3 months.

The rewards for which you receive public recognition and gifts are called 'extrinsic rewards'. This type of reward is highly motivational, particularly when you are starting exercise for the first time or following a long period of inactivity. As you become more involved in exercise you will begin to set 'intrinsic rewards', meaning you meet your target number of sessions in a week or your target number of repetitions of an exercise. The ultimate form of intrinsic reward is that you fully enjoy exercise and doing the exercise is a rewarding experience in itself. There is less public recognition of these achievements and you don't get a prize either; rather, you will take personal pride in your achievements.

Mastery

When designing your exercise programme look for a balance between doing things you feel you are good at and trying new activities. Attempting something new can be motivating, especially if you once associated exercise with unpleasant thoughts and feelings. Keep uppermost that you may find selecting a new exercise or increasing the difficulty (intensity) hard work at first but when you have mastered it there's a great feeling of achievement. This achievement will motivate you to continue exercising and to try more new exercises. The result is a progressive improvement in your fitness and well-being. You are likely to feel downhearted when starting a new exercise as you won't achieve results early in the learning process, but don't give up! Nothing good comes easy, and often the harder the road to success, the greater the feeling of achievement when you have mastered the exercise.

Build in exercise as part of your lifestyle

Plan dedicated periods of time during the day for exercise and prioritise that time above all else. By prioritising exercise you are reinforcing its value as part of daily life and you are building a routine, which is important for maintaining exercise in the long term. On top of that committed time take any opportunity to exercise, however brief – it all counts.

Although I always advocate planned-in exercise, do be flexible and take advantage of other opportunities when they arise. There's no denying that exercising outside during the cold, dark winter nights is very hard, so make sure you take full advantage of the long daylight hours and good weather during the summer. When you visit new places or find yourself in great surroundings, seize the opportunity to get out and exercise while sightseeing. As you become fitter, the prospect of a 3-hour walk through fantastic mountain scenery such as you find in Wales, the Lake District or the Scottish Highlands will

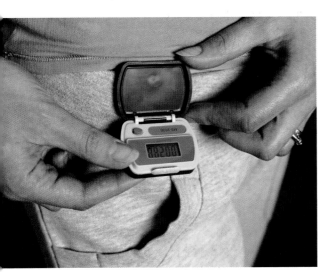

Optimists live longer and cope with stress better. Exercise is enjoyable if you believe it so banish those negative thoughts!

seem all the more enjoyable because it will provide a good endurance session. However, everyday exercise opportunities present themselves: take the stairs, not the lift; build an early-morning walk to the corner shop for a pint of milk into your daily routine. If you are unsure of how much exercise this can give you, buy a pedometer to check the distance you walk per day.

Positive self-talk

Often we have a negative view of exercise. If we constantly repeat those negative thoughts and comments about exercise we can almost hypnotise ourselves into believing that exercise is difficult or unenjoyable. This simply isn't the case, and we need to change that view to positive thinking. Try this simple technique: when you have a negative thought about exercise, change that thought to a positive one and say it out loud. Continue to do this every time you think a negative thought about exercise and soon enough you will start to believe that exercise leads to positive experiences. Keeping hold of positive thoughts about exercise will help to motivate you, and lead to an improved experience in the short term, and make it easier for you maintain your exercise programme in the long term. Remember, exercise is for life, not just for Christmas! Reinforce the message that you really enjoy exercise and before you know it exercise will be an integral part of your life.

5-minute

workouts

There are four main components to fitness: flexibility, muscular strength, muscular (strength) endurance and cardiovascular endurance. It is possible to target two of these elements during exercise that take just 5 minutes – flexibility and strength. Flexibility and strength are important elements of fitness for a number of reasons: they underpin strength and cardiovascular endurance, enhance our quality of life, reduce the risk of injury and help to increase or maintain our muscle mass.

Flexibility is simply the range of motion of a joint, which is governed by the muscles, tendons and ligaments around the joint. In general terms, the greater the range of motion, the easier it is to move. Good flexibility means that routine tasks, such as bending down to tie your shoelaces or reaching up for something on a high shelf, are easier and exercise is more effective. Strength refers to our ability to apply muscular force to move an object. Strength is associated not only with the size of the muscle but also with the way in which we recruit the muscle – that is, ask it to work. In other words, we can be strong without having big muscles.

Why maintaining flexibility and strength is important

Our ability to sustain physical activity for prolonged periods of time requires strong, flexible muscles. The combination of flexibility and strength are important in improving our quality of life by making daily tasks easier to perform: stretching down to the bottom shelf at the supermarket, picking up our children or grandchildren and climbing stairs all require strength and flexibility. If we undertake a variety of strength exercises using the full range of motion, we can expect to improve strength and flexibility simultaneously because the muscles are producing force across the full movement of the joint.

The four components of fitness are interdependent. Without flexibility and strength our endurance capacity would be significantly reduced. Strong, flexible people have a lower incidence of injury. Frailty in later life is too often a direct result of reduced fitness. If we can maintain strength and flexibility we reduce the likelihood of falling in the first place and strong muscles and bones reduce the possibility of fractures. Believe me, it is worth keeping fit throughout your life. Weight-loss programmes often cause a loss in muscle (not fat) mass, yet it is crucial to maintain muscle mass because the bulk of energy is consumed by our muscles. Therefore, if you are to be successful in losing weight, you need to maintain muscle mass to enhance fat loss, which is why I advocate exercise over dieting. The added aesthetic benefit of strength and flexibility exercises is that they develop tone in our muscles, giving our bodies great shape and form.

Workout from head to toe

This range of 5-minute exercises works all major muscle groups and joints. If you complete all the exercises you will improve the flexibility and strength of your entire body. I have grouped the exercises into friendly, easily understood packages, focusing on core strength and stability, bum, tum and thighs, strength and power, and band exercises. With the exception of the flexibility exercises, each exercise is categorised according to difficulty:

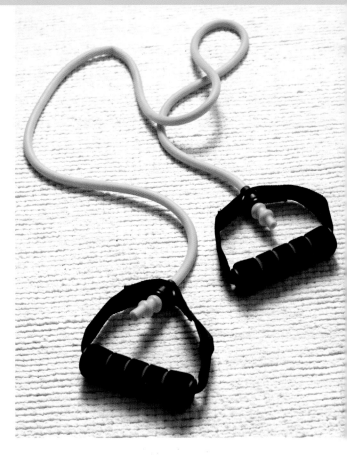

(1) easy, (2) medium and (3) hard, allowing you to progress without increasing the time requirement for the exercises. Each exercise takes approximately 90 seconds to complete, and by selecting three exercises you will be done in 5 minutes and can add another exercise session to your daily and weekly total. Resistance bands (see right) are a great tool to use at home and cost less than £10 from major sports stores. You don't have to go out and buy a professional band, though – a long piece of strong elastic will do the job!

It is important for the core strength and stability, bum, tum and thighs, strength and power, and band exercises that you concentrate on using the full range of motion described in the text accompanying the images. Try not to make the exercise easier by using a smaller range of motion. In addition, apply force slowly and deliberately, concentrating on correct posture and technique. Move up to the next level of difficulty only when you are able easily to complete the level you are currently on. The intensity (difficulty) of the flexibility exercises is set by you; as you improve your flexibility you will be able to increase the range of motion through which you move.

During flexibility exercises it is important that you move *slowly* to a position where you first feel the stretch in the target area and then hold that position for the recommended time. Never push yourself to a position that causes pain. Each flexibility exercise takes around 30 seconds to complete, so think about selecting six to eight flexibility exercises for your 5-minute workout.

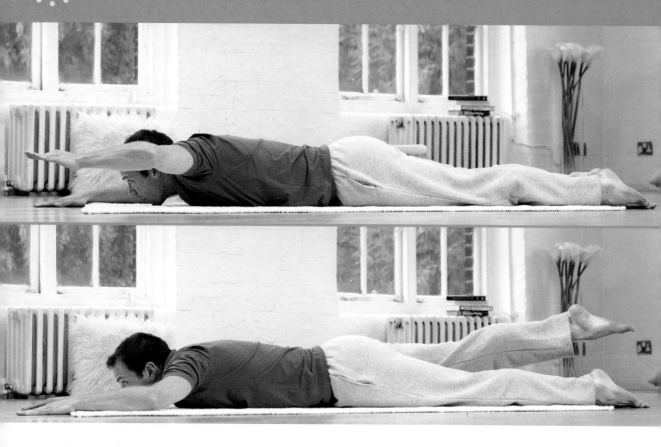

easy

• Lie face down with arms out to the side and elbows bent at 90º

• Lift the left arm and hold for 5 seconds
• Return to the start position
• Repeat for the right leg, left leg and right arm
Repeat 10 times

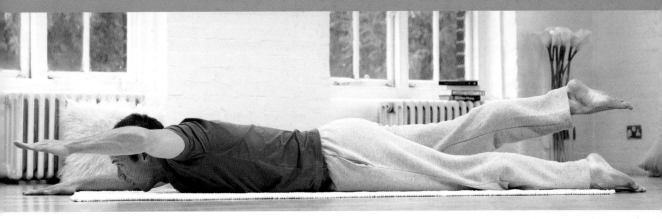

medium

- Lie face down with arms out to the side and elbows bent at 90°
- Lift the left arm and right leg simultaneously and hold for 5 seconds
- Return to the start position

- Lift the right arm and left leg simultaneously and hold for 5 seconds
- Return to the start position
Repeat 20 times

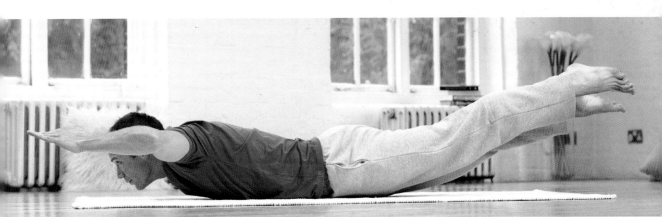

hard

- Lie face down with arms out to the side and elbows bent at 90°
- Lift both arms and both legs simultaneously and hold for 5 seconds

- Return to the start position
Repeat 20 times
Think about length rather than height (stretch out the limbs)

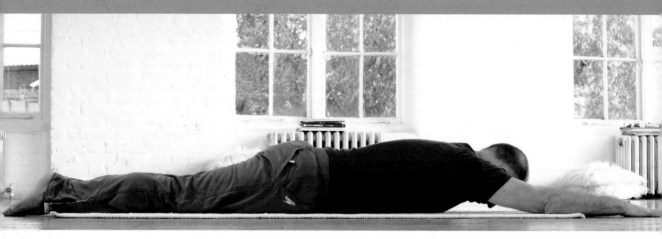

easy

- Lie face down on the floor with your arms extended above your head
- Make your body as long as possible by stretching out your arms and legs

- Hold for 20 seconds
Relax and repeat 3 times

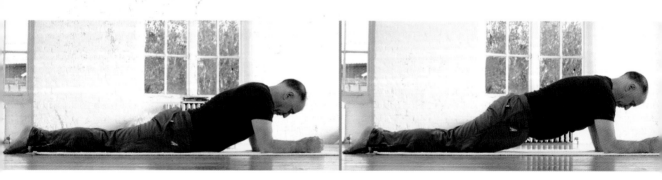

medium

- Lie face down on the floor with your upper body supported by your forearms, elbows beneath your shoulders

- Keeping your knees on the floor, raise your hips, making a straight line between your knees, hips and shoulders
- Hold for 20 seconds
Relax and repeat 3 times

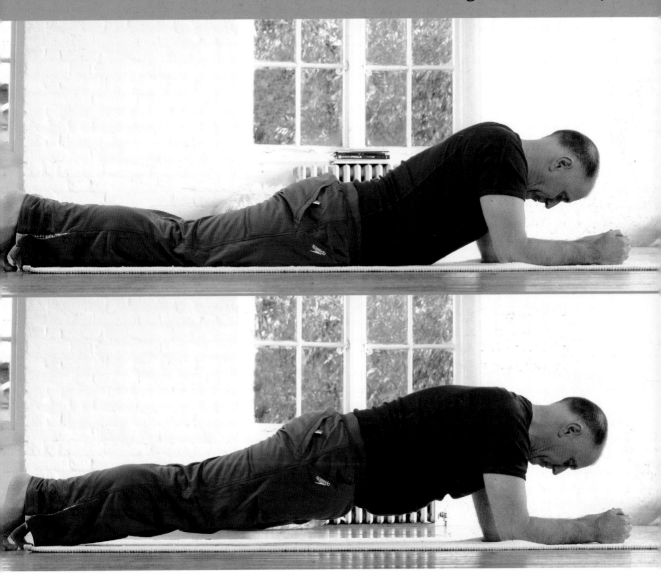

hard

• Lie face-down on the floor with your upper body supported by your forearms, elbows beneath your shoulders

• Raise yourself onto your forearms and the balls of your feet, making a straight line between your heels, hips and shoulders
• Hold for 20 seconds
Relax and repeat 3 times

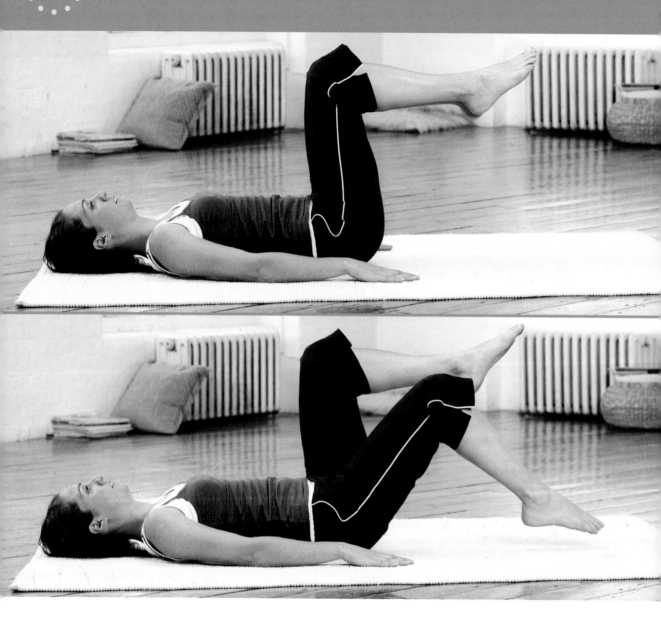

easy

- Lie on your back with your arms by your side
- Pull your knees up and hold them in the air, making a 90° angle at your hips and knees

- Hold one leg in position, then lower the other foot and touch the toe lightly on the floor before returning to the start position
- Repeat with the other leg

Repeat 10 times

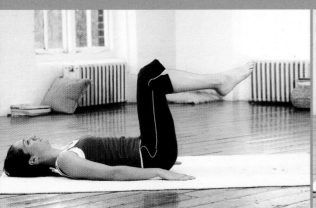 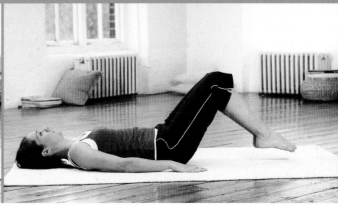

medium

• Lie on your back with your arms by your side
• Pull your knees up and hold them in the air, making a 90° angle at your hips and knees

• Without arching your back, lower both feet and touch the toes lightly on the floor before returning to the start position
Repeat 20 times

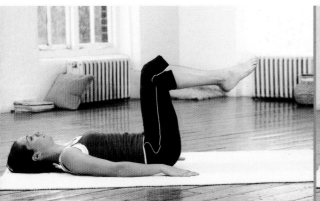 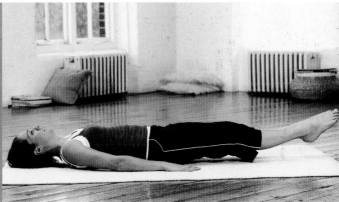

hard

• Lie on your back with your arms by your side
• Pull your knees up and hold them in the air, making a 90° angle at your hips and knees
• Without arching your back, lower both feet, the toes lightly on the floor and, without

sliding the feet along the floor, extend your legs before returning to the start position.
Repeat 10 times

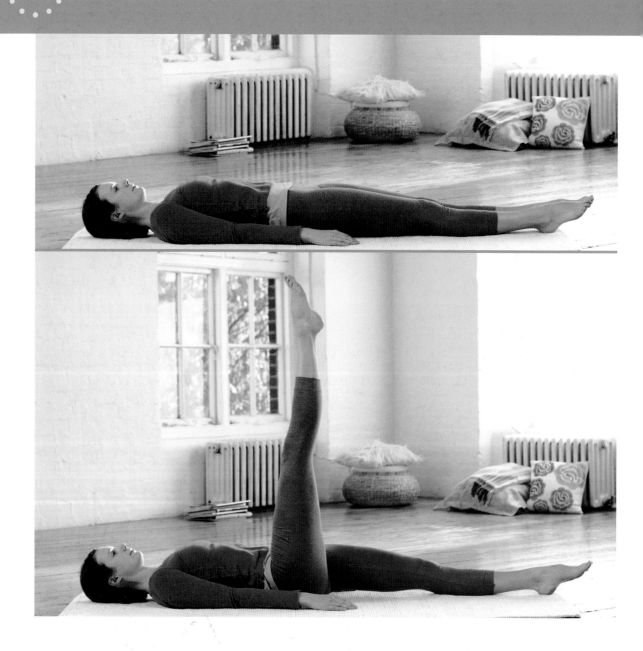

easy

• Lie on your back with your arms by your side and legs fully extended

• Lift the right leg upwards as high as possible, keeping the leg straight
• Lower the leg and repeat for the left leg
Repeat 10 times

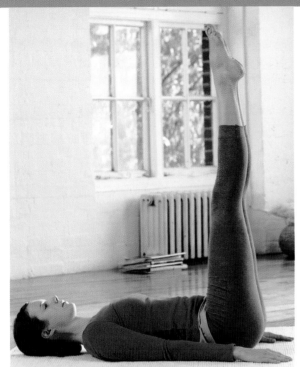

medium

• Lie on your back with your arms by your side and legs fully extended
• Lift both legs in the air, making a 90° angle at your hips
• Maintaining the position of the right leg, lower the left leg until the heel gently touches the ground
• Return to the start position and repeat the exercise, this time lowering the right leg
Repeat 10 times

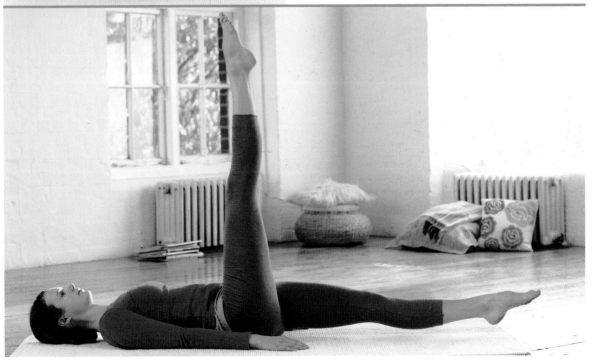

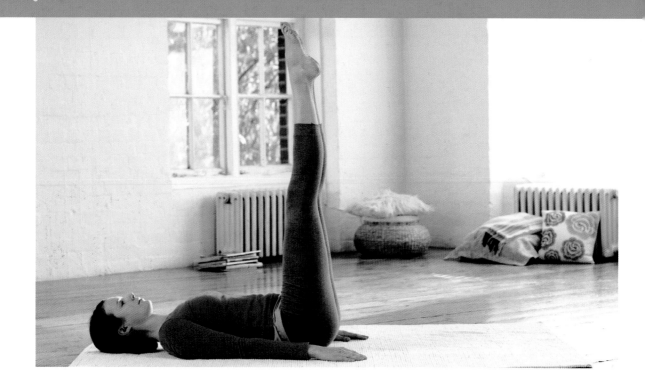

hard

• Lie on your back with your arms by your side and legs fully extended
• Lift both legs in the air, making a 90° angle at your hips

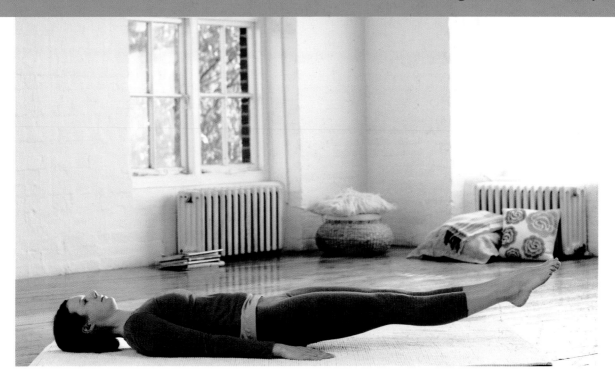

- Lower both legs until the heels gently touch the ground
- Return to the start position

Repeat 10 times

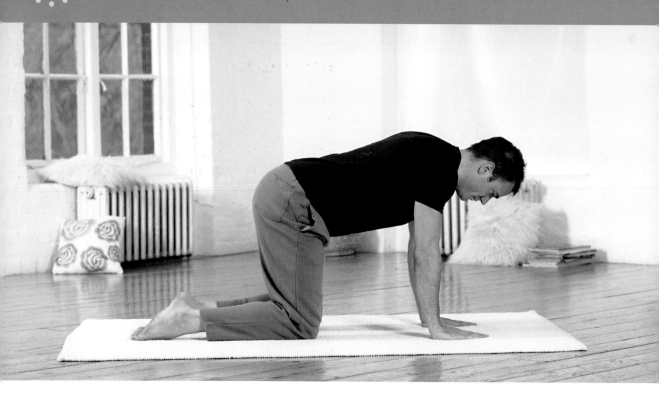

easy

• Position yourself on all fours with your weight evenly distributed between hands and knees and the back long and straight

• Contract all of the muscles surrounding your abdomen, breathing normally, and hold for 20 seconds
Relax and repeat 3 times

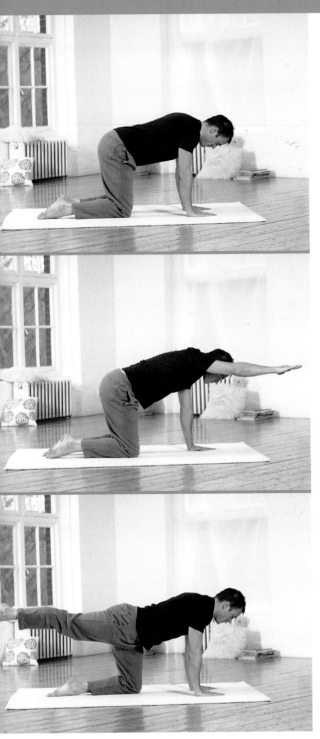

medium

- Position yourself on all fours with your weight evenly distributed between hands and knees and the back long and straight
- Contract all of the muscles surrounding your abdomen and breathe normally
- Keeping the position, extend your right arm directly forwards and hold for 5 seconds
- Return to the start position
- Without collapsing the arms, extend your right leg directly backwards to form a straight line from heel to knee to bum to shoulder and hold for 5 seconds
- Return to the start position
- Repeat the above for the left arm and left leg

Relax and repeat 3 times

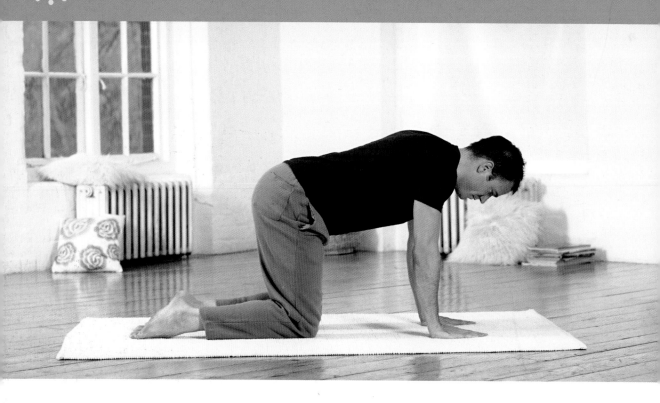

hard

• Position yourself on all fours with your weight evenly distributed between hands and knees and the back long and straight
• Contract all of the muscles surrounding your abdomen and breathe normally

• Without collapsing the arms extend, your left leg directly backwards and your right arm directly forwards and hold for 5 seconds
• Return to the start position
• Repeat the above for the right leg and left arm
Relax and repeat 5 times

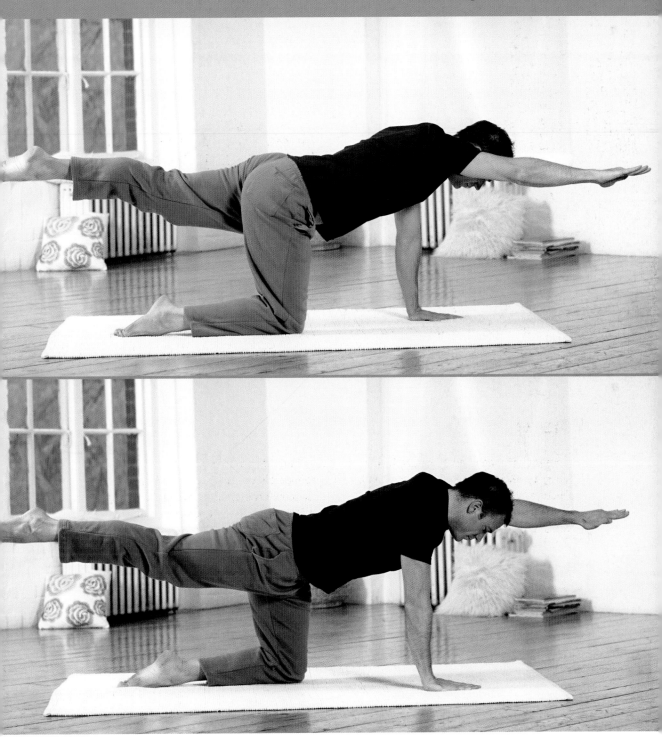

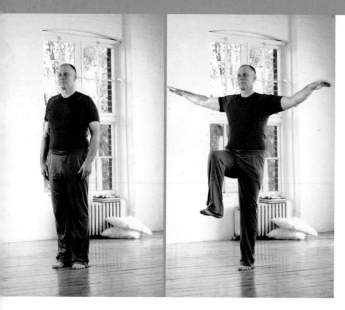

easy

• Stand upright with feet shoulder-width apart and looking forwards
• With your eyes open and using your arms for balance, stand on one leg and hold for 15 seconds
• Return to the start position and repeat the above for the other leg
Repeat 3 times

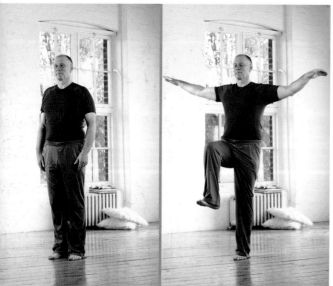

medium

• Stand upright with feet shoulder-width apart and looking forwards
• With your eyes closed and using your arms for balance, stand on one leg and hold for 15 seconds
• Return to the start position and repeat the above for the other leg
Repeat 3 times

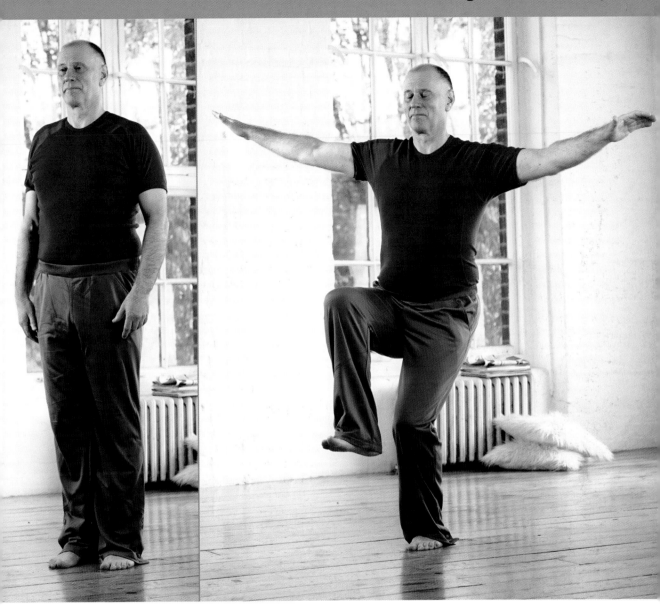

hard

• Stand upright with feet shoulder-width apart and looking forwards
• With your eyes closed and using your arms for balance, stand on one leg

• Squat down as low as possible and return to the start position
• Repeat the above for the other leg
Repeat 10 times

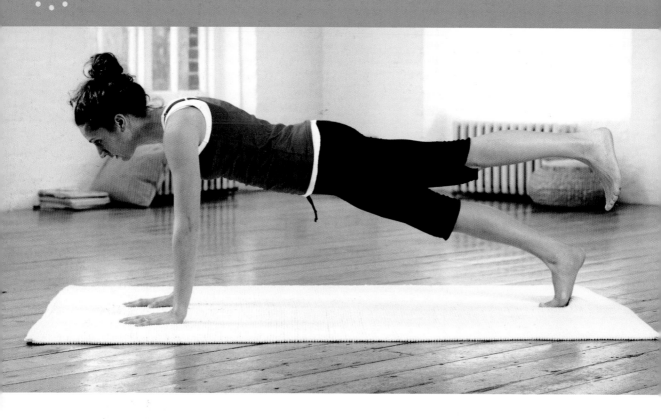

easy

• In the press-up position, form a straight line from your head to your knees
• Breathe out, extend the left leg and lift it, making a straight line from hip to knee to ankle

Lower to the start position and repeat 10 times on each leg

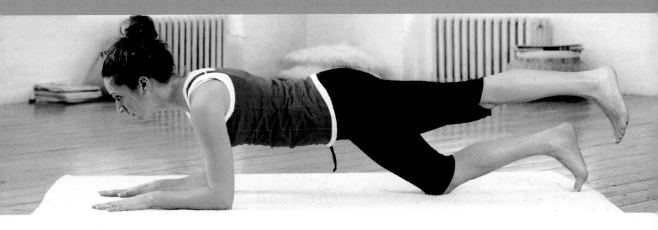

medium

- Lie face down with your forearms on the floor, palms facing down
- Raise yourself onto your forearms and knees, keeping the lower leg on the floor

- Breathe out and extend the left leg, making a straight line from hip to knee to ankle

Lower to the start position and repeat 10 times on each leg

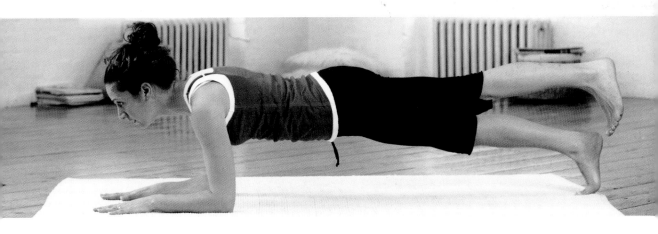

hard

- Lie face down, with your forearms on the floor, palms facing down and level with the top of your head
- Raise yourself onto your forearms and the balls of your feet, making a straight line

between your heels, hips and shoulders
- Breathe out and extend the left leg, making a straight line from shoulder to hip to ankle

Lower to the start position and repeat 10 times on each leg

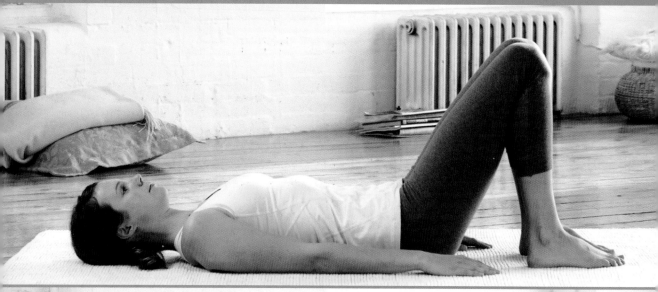

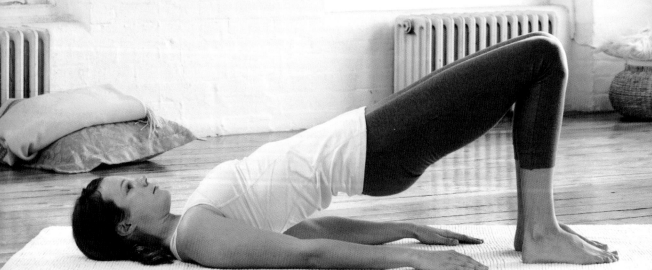

easy

• Lie on your back, hands by your side and knees bent with feet shoulder-width apart

• Roll your hips to the ceiling until you are resting on your shoulders with a straight line from shoulders to hips to knees and hold for 10 seconds
Return to start position and repeat 5 times

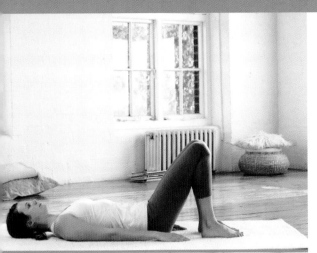

medium

- Lie on your back, hands by your side and knees bent with feet shoulder-width apart
- Roll your hips to the ceiling until you are resting on your shoulders with a straight line from shoulders to hips to knees
- In that position extend one leg, raise it with your knees at the same height and hold for 10 seconds

Return to the start position and repeat 10 times, alternating legs

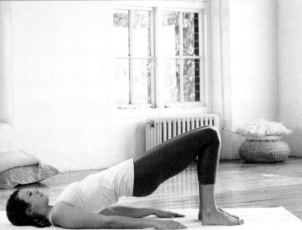

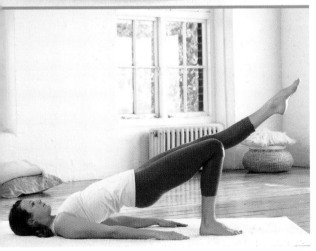

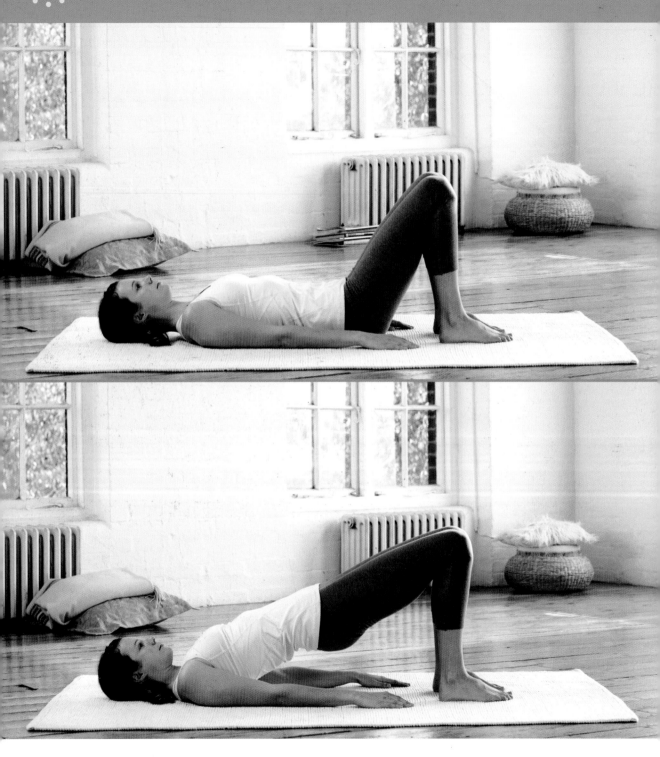

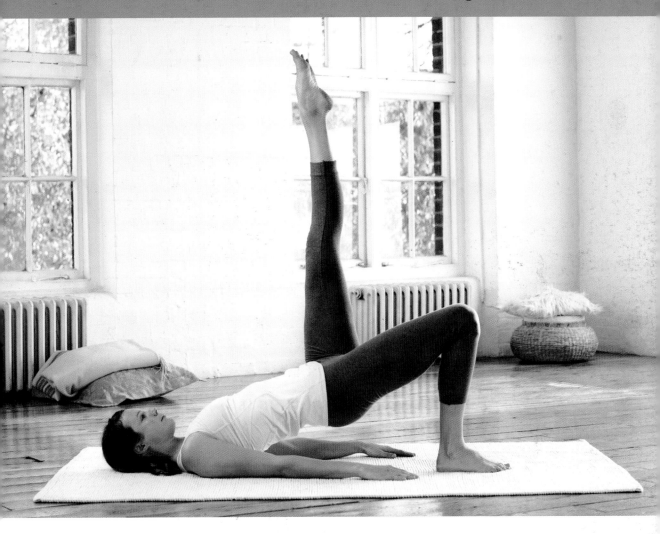

hard

• Lie on your back, hands by your side and knees bent with feet shoulder-width apart
• Roll your hips to the ceiling until you are resting on your shoulders with a straight line from shoulders to hips to knees

• In that position extend one leg, raise it to the ceiling and hold for 10 seconds
Return to the start position and repeat 10 times, alternating legs

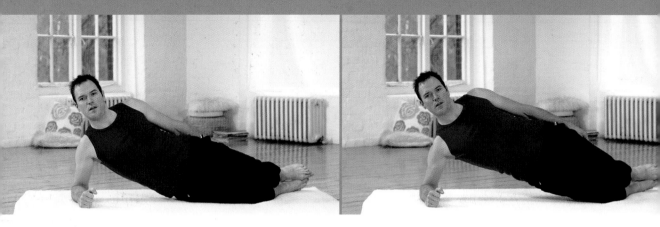

easy

• Sit on your right hip with knees bent and resting on your right elbow
• Without collapsing the arm, lift the hip to the ceiling, keeping the knees on the floor and

making a straight line from shoulder to hip to knee; hold for 10 seconds
Return to start position and repeat 3 times
• Roll over and repeat for the left hip

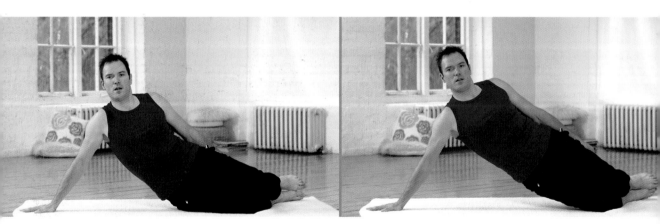

medium

• Sit on your right hip with knees bent and right arm extended under your right shoulder
• Without collapsing the arm, lift the hip to the ceiling, keeping your knees on the floor and

making a straight line from shoulder to hip to ankle; hold for 10 seconds
Return to start position and repeat 3 times
• Roll over and repeat for the left hip

66   GET FIT not fat

Side raise
Core strength and stability

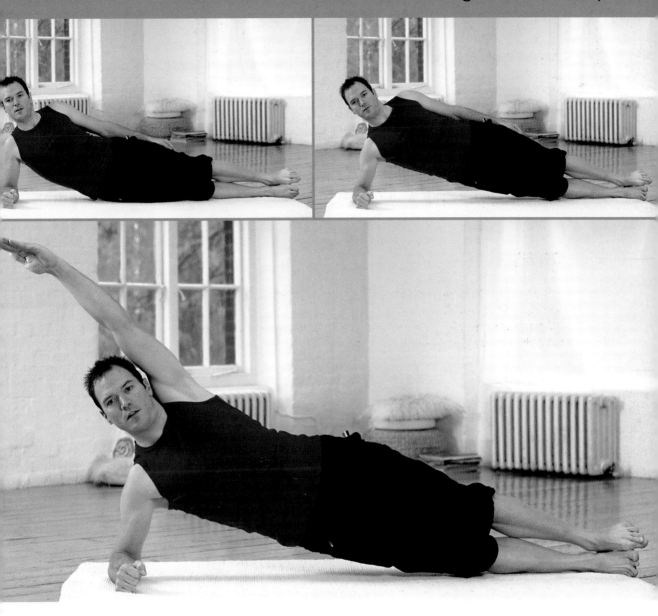

hard

- Sit on your right hip with legs straight and resting on your right elbow
- Without collapsing the arm, lift the hips, making a straight line from shoulder to ankle
- Extend your left arm above your head and hold for 10 seconds

Return to start position and repeat 3 times

- Roll over and repeat for the left hip

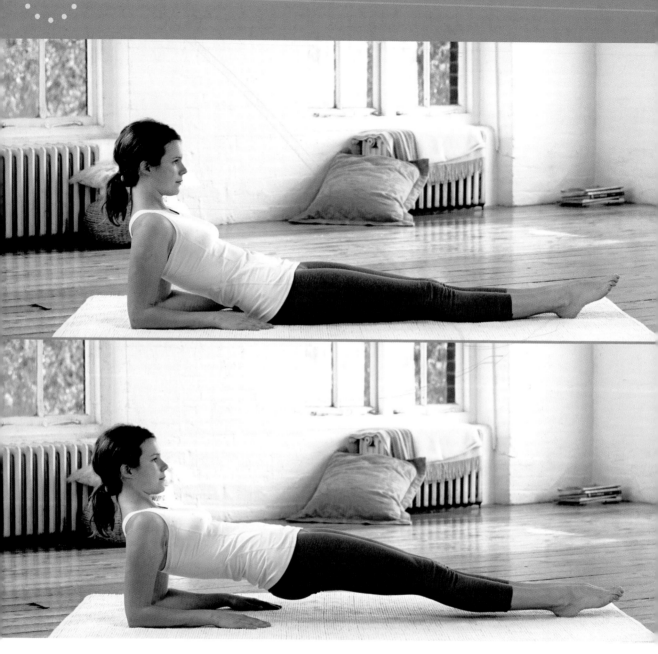

easy

• Sit on the floor with your upper body resting on your elbows and legs out straight
• Lift your hips to the ceiling, making a straight line from shoulders to hips to ankles, and hold for 10 seconds

Return to start position and repeat 5 times

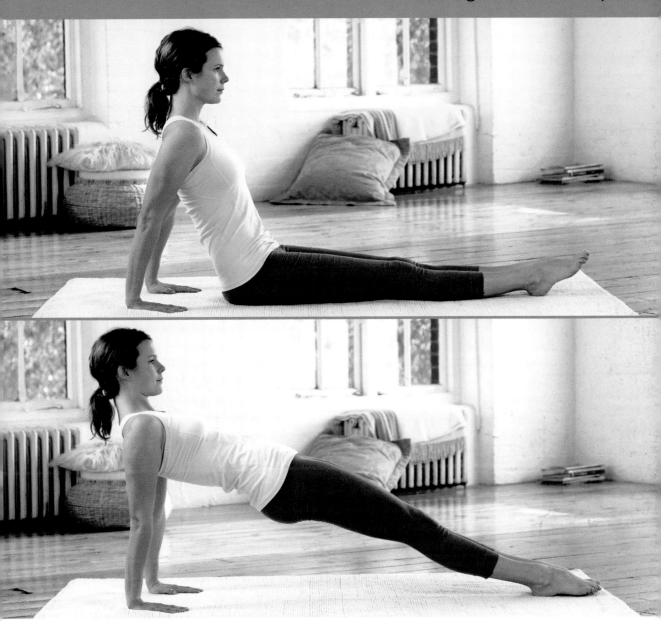

medium

• Sit on the floor with your arms extended behind, your upper body resting on your hands
• Lift your hips to the ceiling, making a straight line from shoulders to hips to ankles, and hold for 10 seconds

Return to start position and repeat 5 times

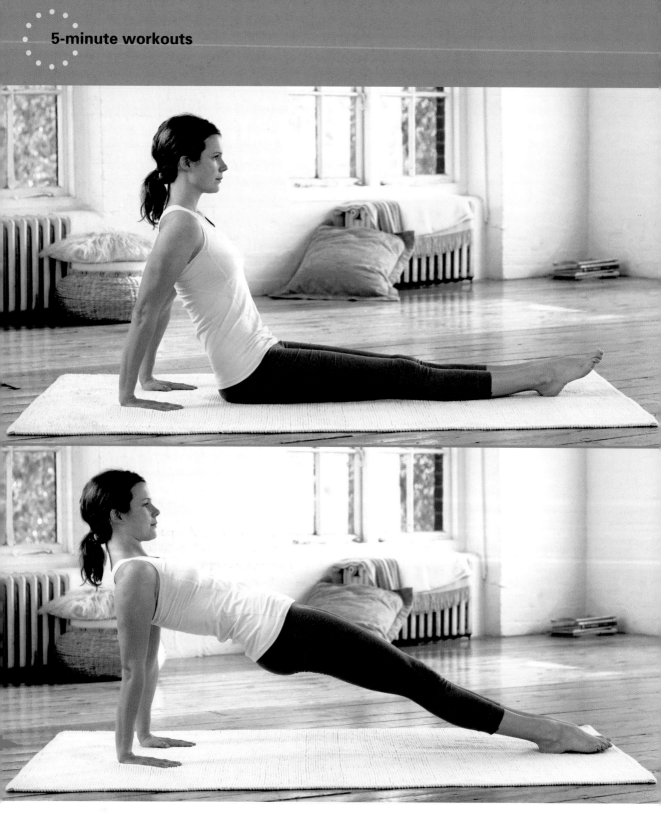

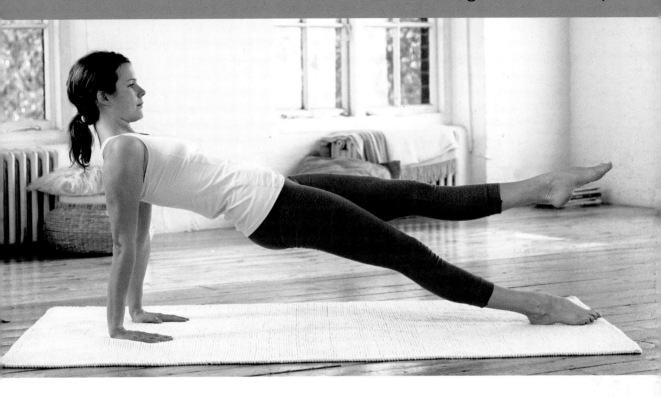

hard

- Sit on the floor with your arms extended behind, your upper body resting on your hands, and your legs out straight
- Lift your hips to the ceiling making a straight line from shoulders to hips to ankles

- In that position lift your left leg to the same height as your hip and hold for 10 seconds
- Repeat with your right leg

Return to the start position and repeat 3 times

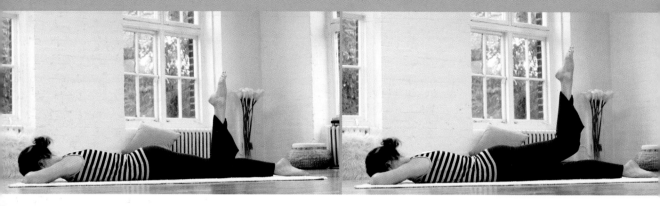

easy

- Lie face down. Draw the navel towards the back and tense the legs and bottom
- Bend the left leg at the knee at 90°, raise the left thigh off the floor while keeping the hips in contact with the floor and hold for 5 seconds
- Return to the start position and change legs
Repeat 20 times

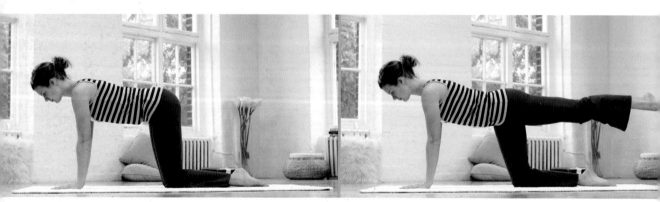

medium

- Start on all fours with your weight evenly distributed. Without collapsing the arms, extend the left leg directly backwards to form a straight line from heel to knee to bum to shoulder and hold for 5 seconds
- Return to the start position and change legs
Repeat 20 times

hard

• Start on all fours with your weight evenly distributed. Without collapsing the arms, lift the left leg directly upwards. Imagine your toes are being pulled by a string straight up to the ceiling and hold for 5 seconds
• Return to the start position and change legs
Repeat 20 times

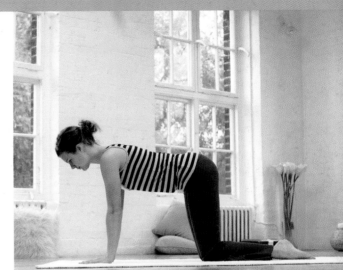

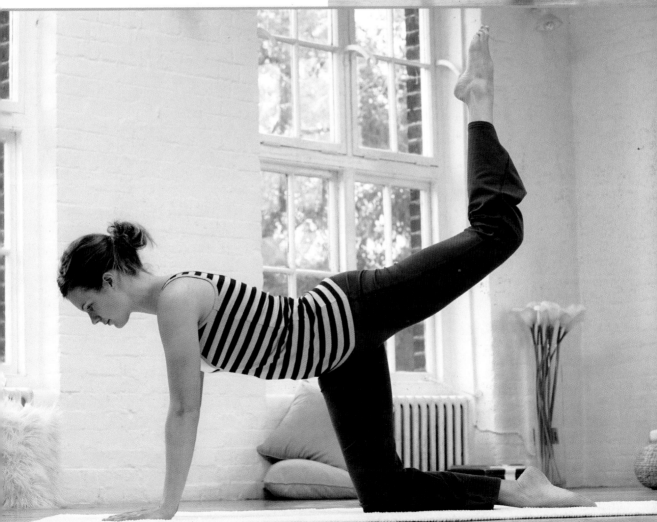

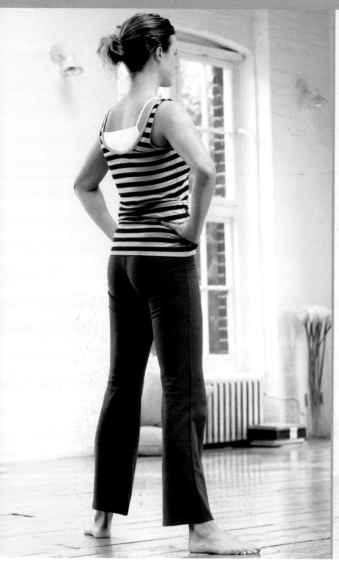 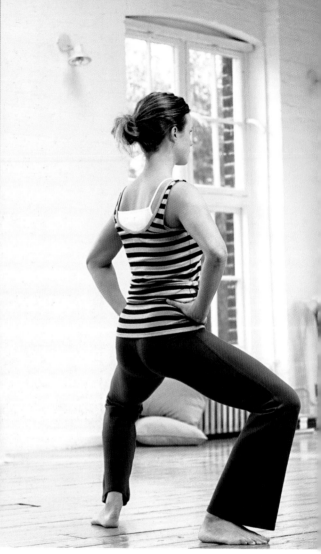

easy

• Stand with the legs just more than
shoulder-width apart, with feet turned out
and hands on hips

• Squat down, keeping your back straight and
looking forwards
• Return to the start position
Repeat 20 times

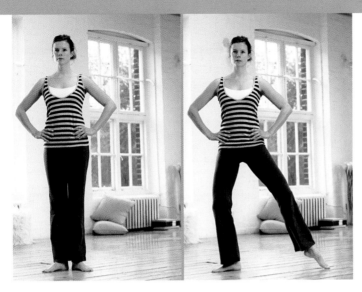

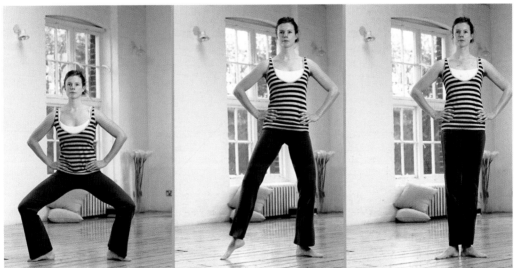

medium

- Stand with legs together
- Take a large step to the left
- Squat down with feet turned out, keeping your back straight and looking forwards

- Step to the right, returning to a standing position
- Repeat the steps above, moving to the right
Repeat 20 times

hard

• Stand with the legs just more than shoulder-width apart, with feet turned out and hands on hips
• Squat down, keeping your back straight and looking forwards
• Jump upwards, as high as possible, and on landing move immediately to the squat position
Repeat 20 times

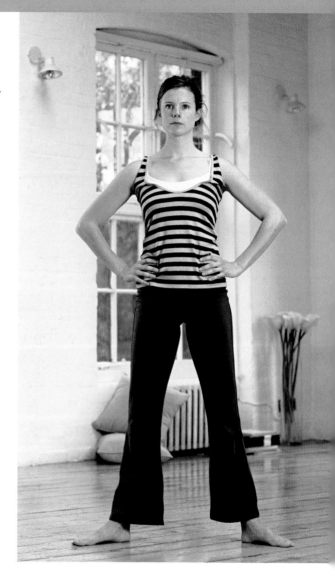

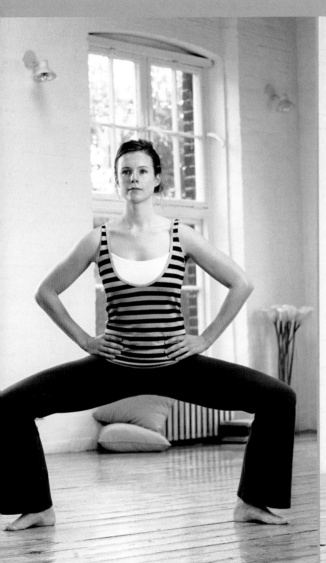 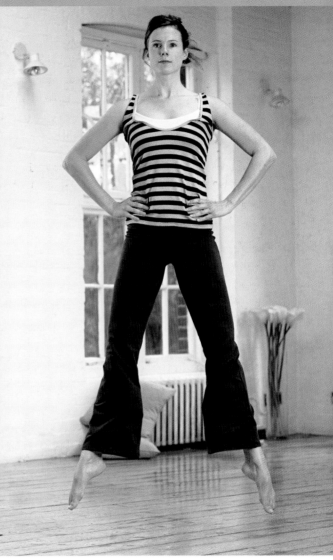

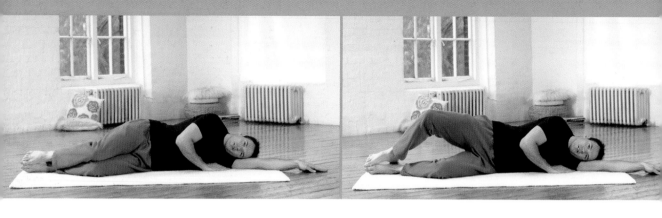

easy

• Lie on your left side with your lower arm extended above your head. Keep the legs together, bent at 45°, making a straight line from shoulders to hips to feet

• Keeping the feet together, lift the upper knee as high as possible
• Return to the start position
Repeat 20 times
• Turn over and repeat with the opposite leg

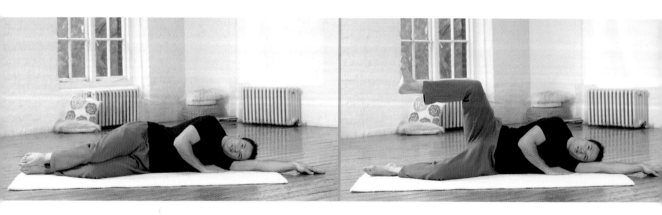

medium

• Lie on your left side with your lower arm extended above your head. Keep the legs together, bent at 45°, making a straight line from shoulders to hips to feet

• Lift the upper knee as high as possible, keeping the lower leg on the floor
• Return to the start position
Repeat 20 times
• Turn over and repeat with the opposite leg

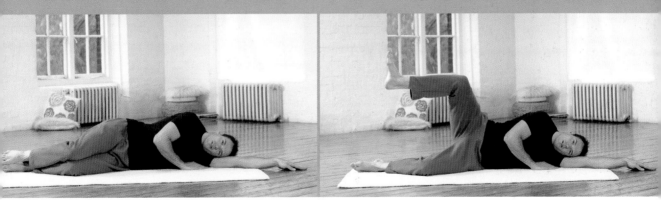

hard

• Lie on your left side with your lower arm extended above your head. Keep the legs together, bent at 45°, making a straight line from shoulders to hips to feet
• Lift the upper knee as high as possible, keeping the lower leg on the floor

• Extend the leg while maintaining the knee at the same height
• Return to the start position
Repeat 20 times
• Turn over and repeat with the opposite leg

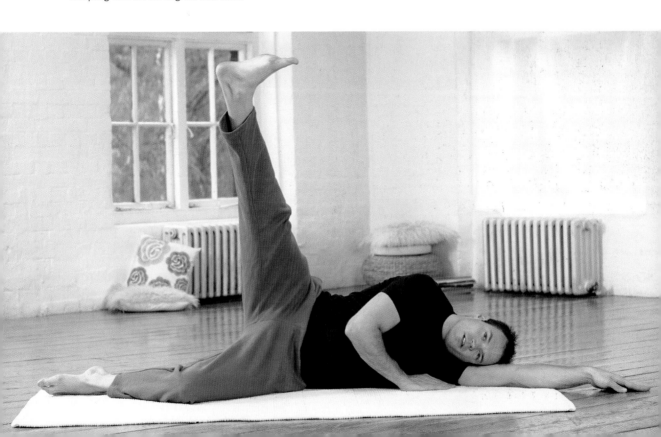

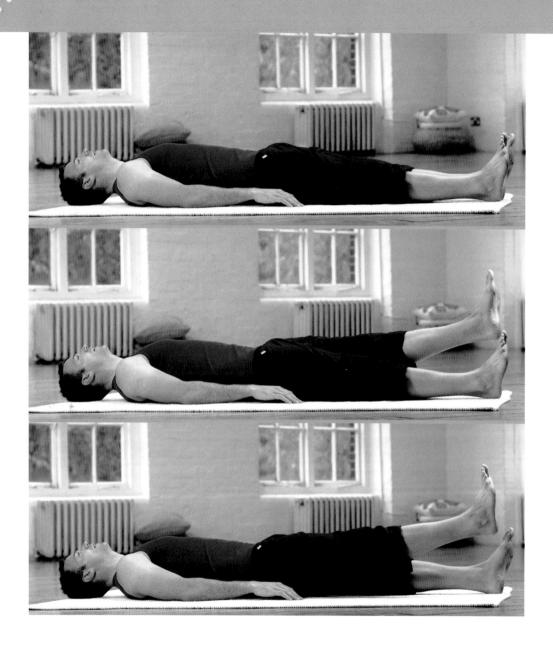

easy

• Lie on your back with your arms by your side
• Without arching the back, lift one leg
20–30cm off the floor and hold for 5 seconds

• Return to the start position and repeat with
the other leg
Repeat 20 times

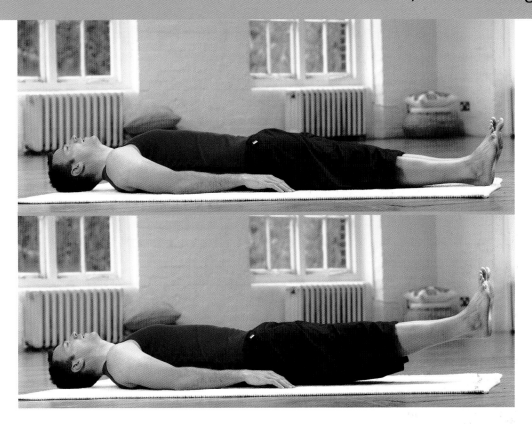

medium

- Lie on your back with your arms by your side
- Without arching the back, lift both legs 20–30cm off the floor and hold for 5 seconds
- Return to the start position

Repeat 20 times

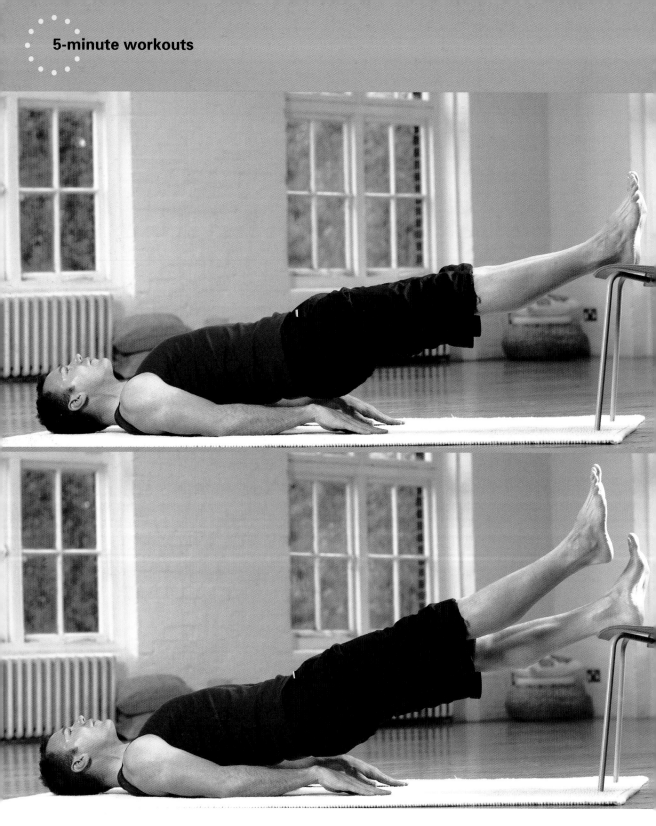

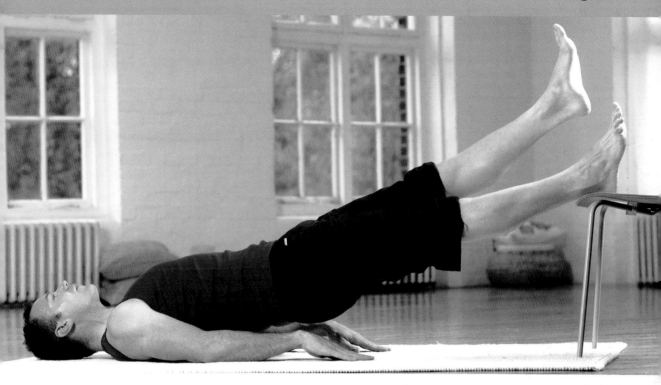

hard

- Lie on your back with your arms by your side
- Place both heels on a chair and lift your hips to form a straight line from shoulders to hips to ankles

- Keeping the back straight, lift one leg 20–30cm off the chair and hold for 5 seconds
- Return to the start position and repeat with the other leg
Repeat 20 times

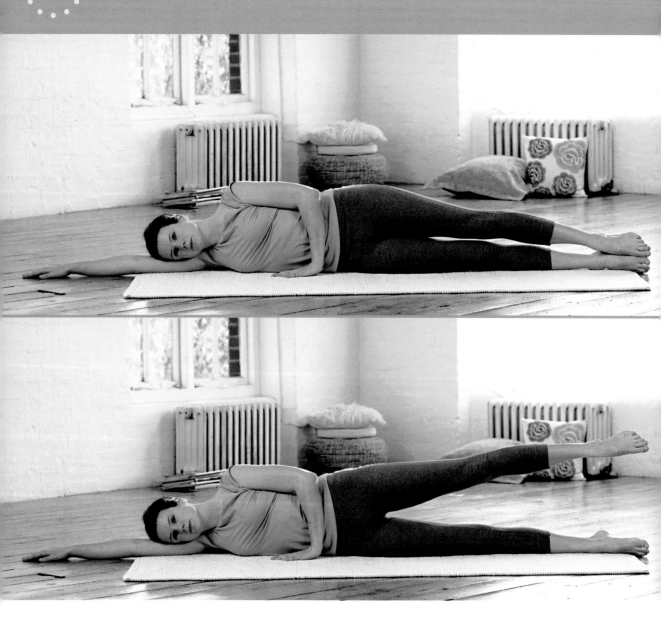

easy

- Lie on your side with the lower arm extended above your head and the upper arm supporting the body
- Straighten the body and, without falling forwards or backwards, lift your upper leg by about 30cm, keeping the leg straight
- Return to the start position
Repeat 10 times
- Turn over and repeat with the other leg

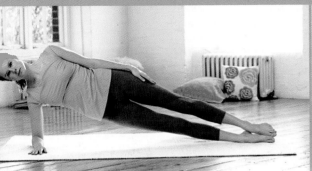 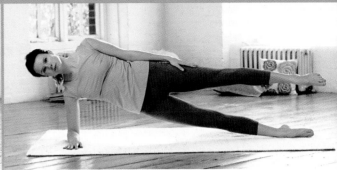

medium

- Lie on your side, and, keeping your upper arm resting on your side, lean on your lower arm and lift the hip upwards to form a straight line from shoulders to hips to feet

- Without falling forwards or backwards, lift your upper leg by about 30cm, keeping the leg straight
- Return to the start position
Repeat 10 times
- Turn over and repeat with the other leg

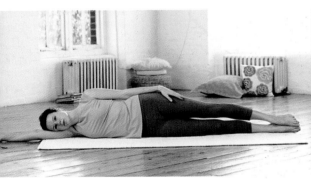 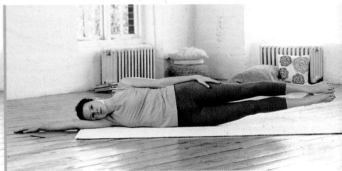

hard

- Lie on your side with the lower arm extended above your head and the upper arm resting on your side
- Straighten the body and, without falling forwards or backwards, lift both legs by about

20cm, keeping the legs straight
- Return to the start position
Repeat 10 times
- Turn over and repeat with the other leg

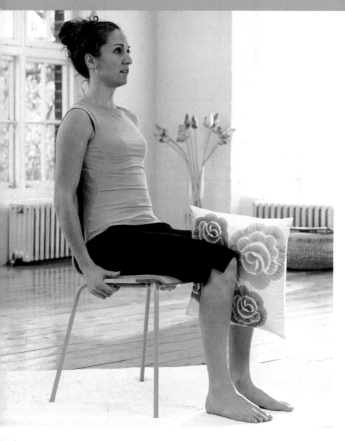

easy

• Sit on a chair and place a firm cushion between your knees
• Squeeze your knees together and hold for 5 seconds
Relax and repeat 20 times

medium

• Lie on the floor with the legs bent at 90° and place a firm cushion between your knees
• Lift your legs with your thighs vertical and your lower legs parallel with the floor
• Squeeze your knees together and hold for 5 seconds
Relax and repeat 20 times

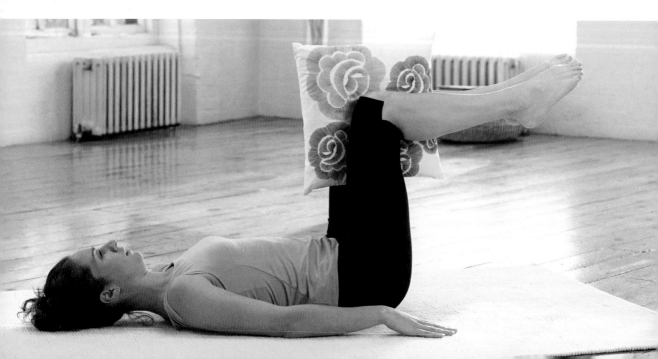

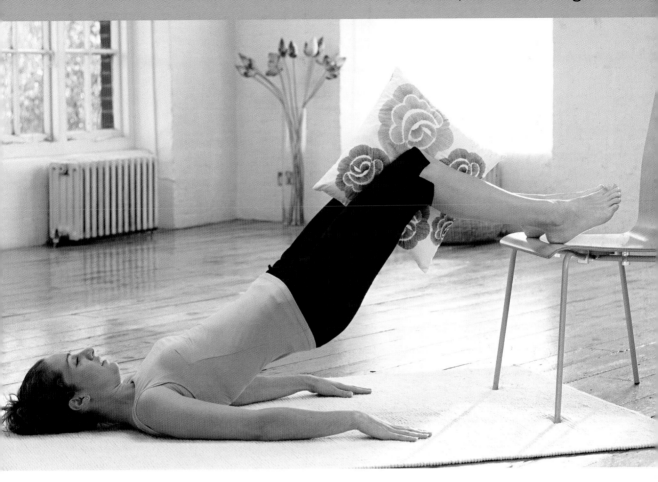

hard

- Lie on your back with your arms by your sides
- Place both heels on a chair and, with your knees bent at 90°, lift your hips to form a straight line from shoulders to hips to ankles

- Place a firm cushion between your knees
- Squeeze your knees together and hold for 5 seconds
Relax and repeat 20 times

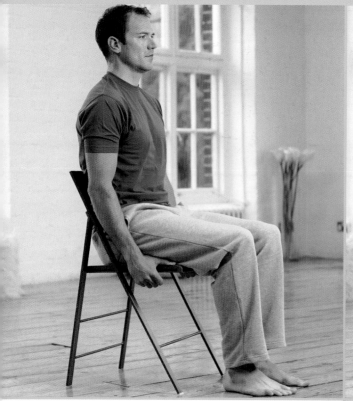

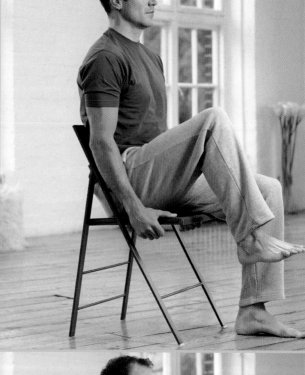

easy

- Sit on a chair with your back straight and looking forwards
- Lift one knee towards the chest
- Return to the start position
- Change legs
Repeat 20 times

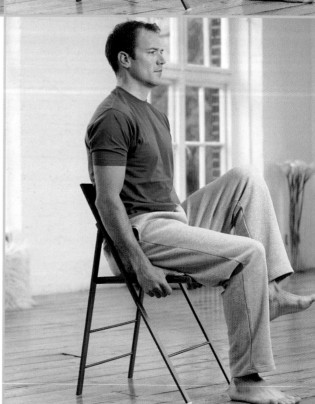

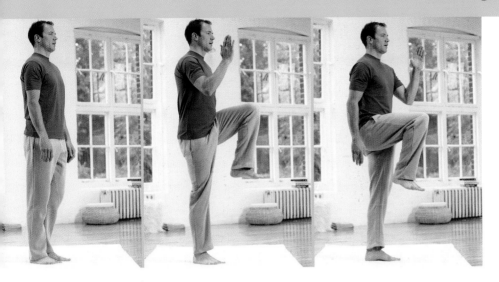

medium

- Stand tall with feet shoulder-width apart
- Lift one leg towards the chest and raise the opposite arm, mimicking a running action

- Alternate legs and arms
Repeat 20 times

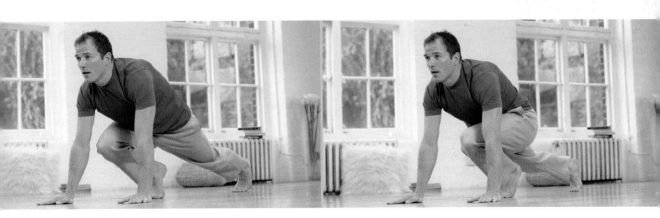

hard

- Start in the push-up position with your weight evenly distributed
- Without collapsing the arms, lift one knee to the chest

- Return to the start position
- Change legs
Repeat 20 times

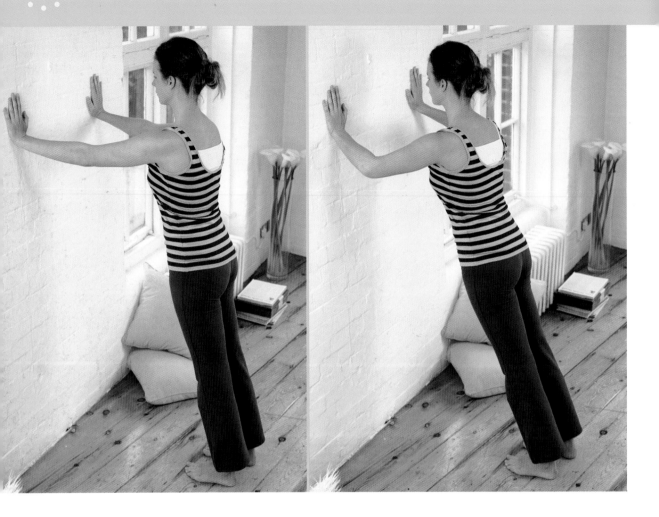

easy

• Stand with feet together about 60cm from a wall, arms outstretched and hands placed on the wall, shoulder-width apart
• Form a straight line from your head to your toes

• Lower your body to the wall
• When the arms are at 90°, pause and straighten the arms
Repeat 20 times

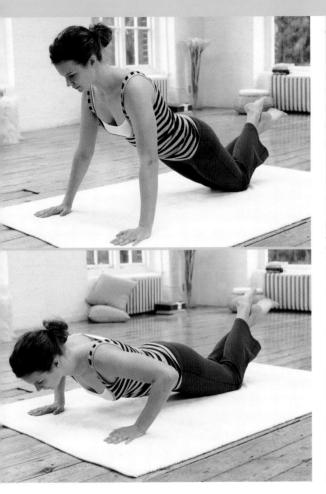

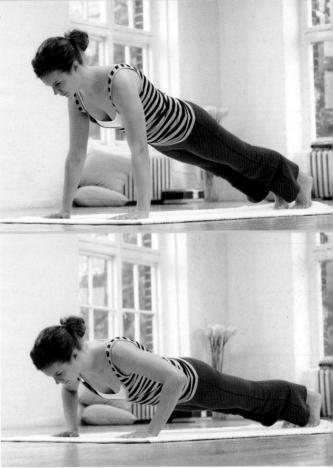

medium

- Start with legs bent and knees together on the floor and arms outstretched with hands shoulder-width apart on the floor
- Form a straight line from your head to your knees
- Lower your body to the floor
- When the arms are at 90°, pause and straighten the arms

Repeat 20 times

hard

- Start with legs straight and feet together on the floor and arms outstretched with hands shoulder-width apart on the floor
- Form a straight line from your head to your knees
- Lower your body to the floor
- When the arms are at 90°, pause and straighten the arms

Repeat 20 times

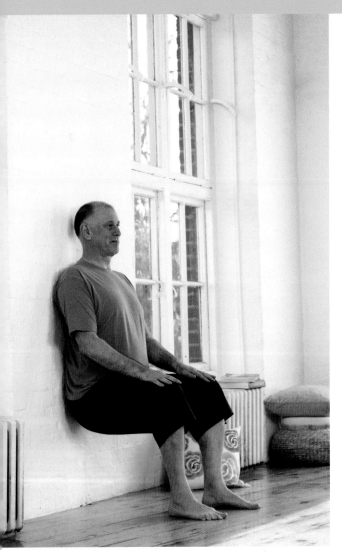

easy

• Stand against a wall with feet shoulder-width apart and hands on the front of your thighs

• Take a small step forwards and, keeping the back straight and looking forwards, bend the legs to 90° and rest your back against the wall

• Hold for 15 seconds

• Stand up and rest for 15 seconds

Repeat 3 times

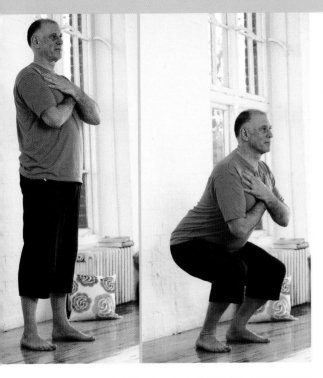

medium

- Stand with feet shoulder-width apart and arms crossed on your chest
- Keeping the back straight and looking forwards, bend the legs to 90°
- Return to the start position

Repeat 20 times

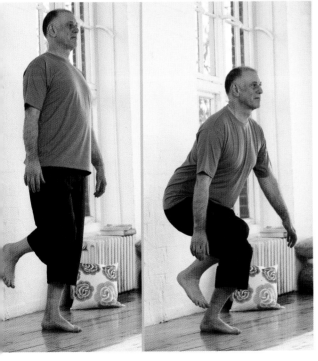

hard

- Stand with feet shoulder-width apart and arms by your sides
- Keeping the back straight and looking forwards, bend one leg to 90° while using the opposite leg and arms to stabilise the body
- Return to the start position

Repeat 10 times

- Repeat with the other leg

easy

• Stand upright with feet shoulder-width apart and looking forwards
• Take a large step forwards
• Keeping the upper body upright and looking forwards, bend the front leg to 90° so that the knee is over the foot
• Return to the start position
• Repeat with the other leg
Repeat 10 times

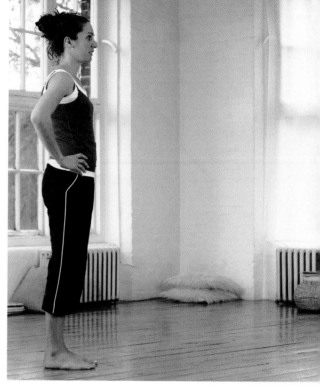

medium

• Stand upright with feet shoulder-width apart and looking forwards
• Take a large step forwards and immediately bend the front leg to 90° so that the knee is over the foot, keeping the upper body upright and looking forwards
• Repeat with the other leg
Repeat 10 times

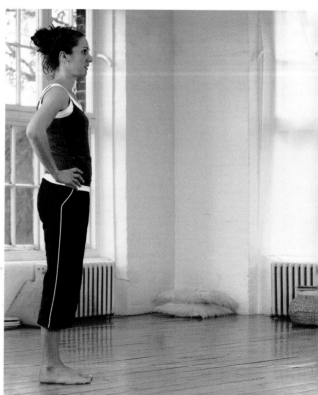

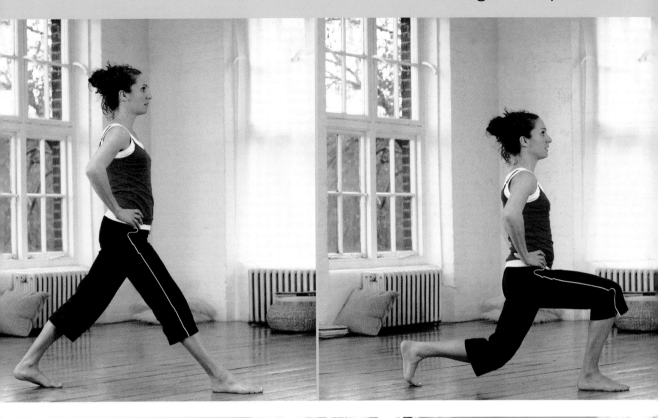

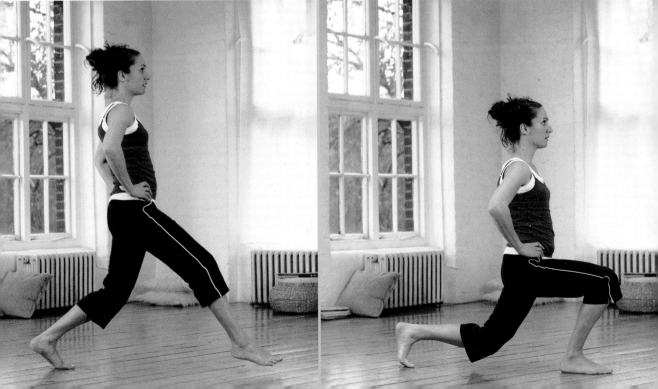

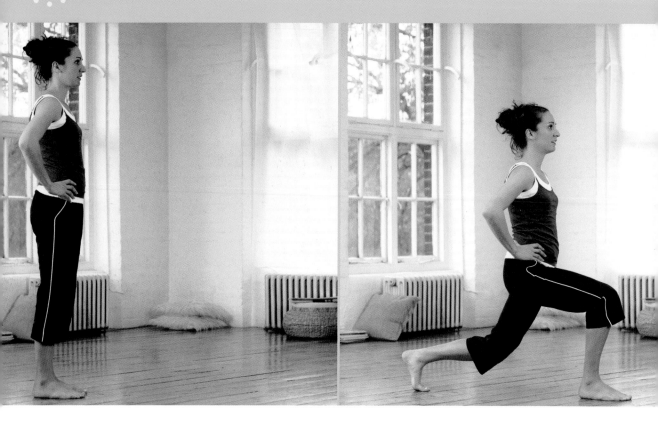

hard

• Stand upright with feet shoulder-width apart and looking forwards
• Take a large step forwards
• Keeping the upper body upright and looking forwards bend the front leg to 90° so that the knee is over the foot

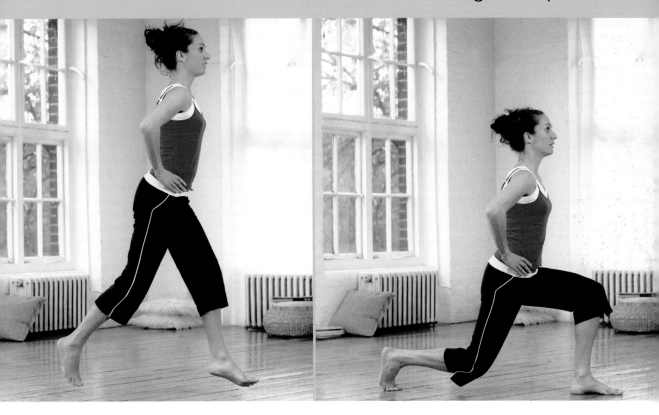

• From the lunge position drive the body upwards using the legs and while in the air swap legs and return to the lunge position with the other leg leading
Repeat 10 times for each leg

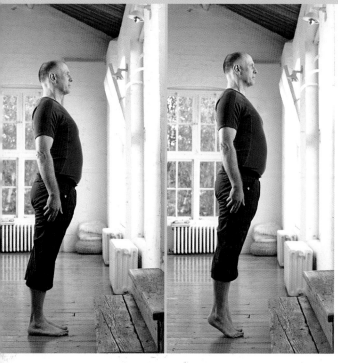

easy

• Stand upright with feet shoulder-width apart and looking forwards
• Extend both ankles to stand on tip toes
• Return to the start position
Repeat 20 times

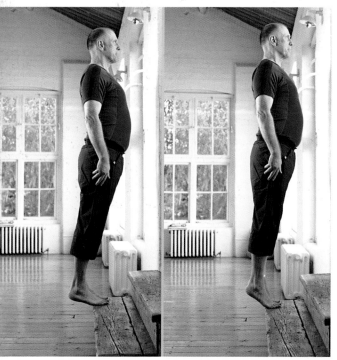

medium

• With the balls of the feet placed on the edge of a step, stand upright with feet shoulder-width apart and looking forwards
• Drop the ankles down and then extend both ankles to stand on tip toes
• Return to the start position
Repeat 20 times

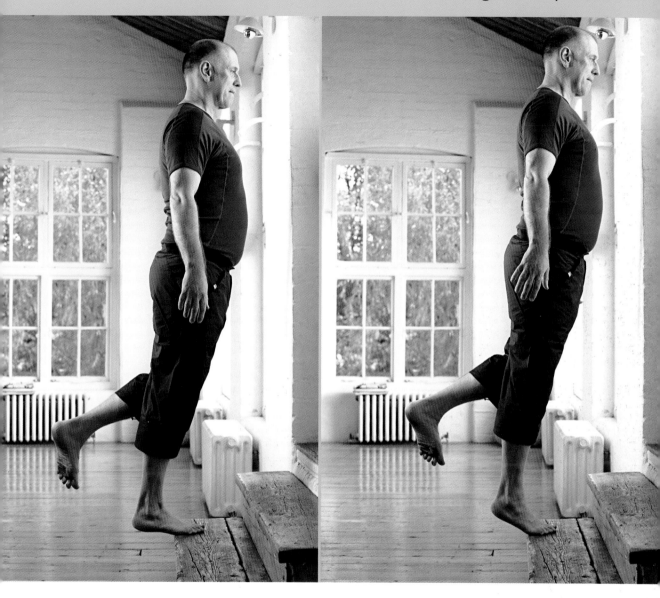

hard

• With the balls of the feet placed on the edge of a step, stand upright with feet shoulder-width apart and looking forwards (use a wall to stabilise the body if required)

• On one leg drop the ankle down and then extend the ankle to stand on tip toes
• Return to the start position
Repeat 20 times
• Repeat with the other leg

easy

- Stand upright with feet shoulder-width apart and looking forwards
- Turn one foot out so that it is at 90° to the other foot
- Take a large step to the side of the foot facing outwards
- Keeping the upper body upright, bend the leading leg to 90° so that the knee is over the foot
- Return to the start position
- Repeat with the other leg

Repeat 10 times

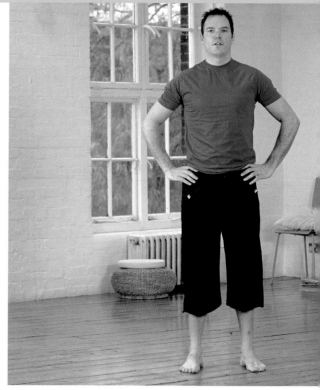

medium

- Stand upright with feet shoulder-width apart and looking forwards
- Turn one foot out so that it is at 90° to the other foot
- Take a large step to the side of the foot facing outwards
- Keeping the upper body upright, immediately bend the leading leg to 90° so that the knee is over the foot
- Return to the start position
- Repeat with the other leg

Repeat 10 times

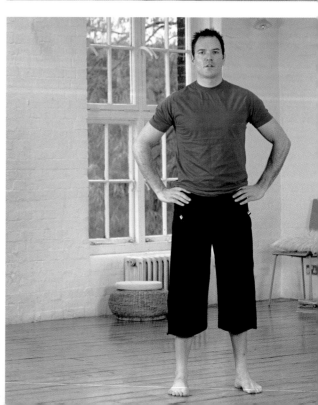

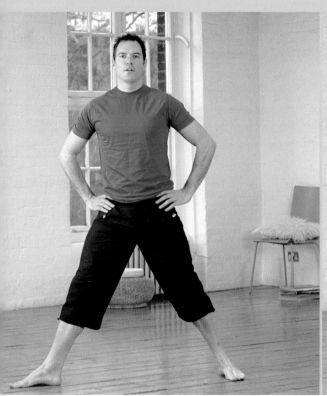
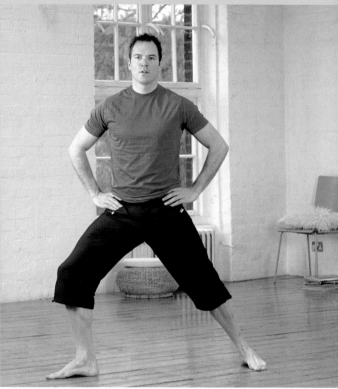
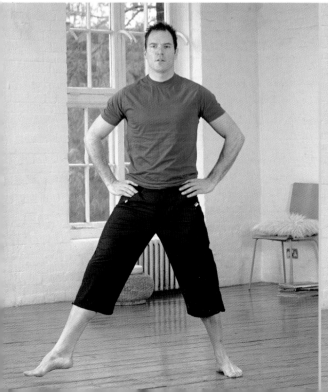
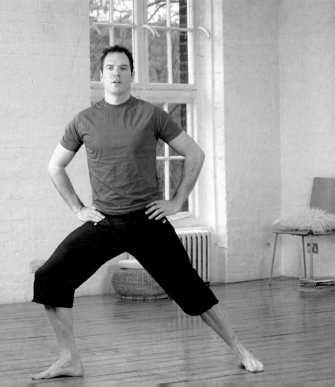

hard

• Stand upright with feet shoulder-width apart and looking forwards
• Turn one foot out so that it is at 90° to the other foot
• Take a large step to the side of the foot facing outwards
• Keeping the upper body upright, immediately bend the leading leg to 90° so that the knee is over the foot
• From the lunge position drive the body upwards using the legs and while in the air rotate the body to look in the opposite direction and return to the lunge position with the other leg leading
Repeat 10 times for each leg

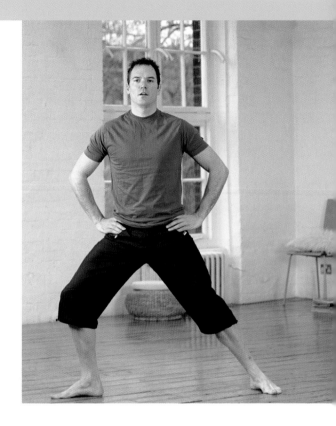

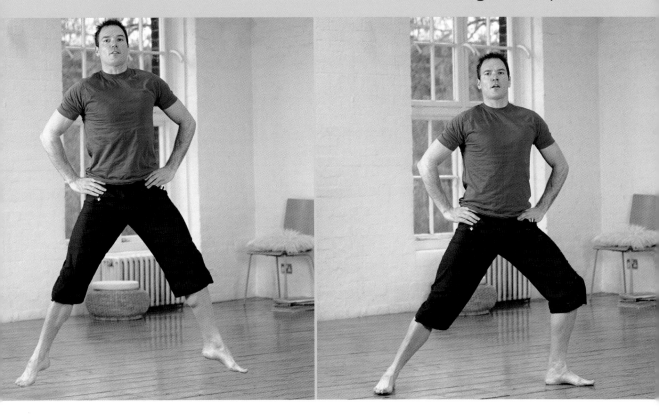

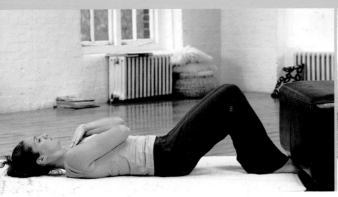 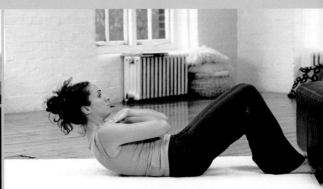

easy

- Lie flat on your back with your legs bent, then tuck your feet under a secure chair, table or door
- Place your hands across your chest, each touching the opposite shoulder

- Lift your head and shoulders towards your knees
- Lift your shoulders about 20cm off the floor and return slowly to the start position
Repeat 20 times

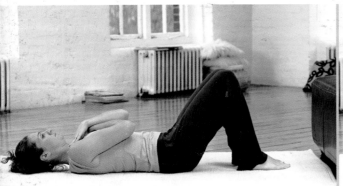 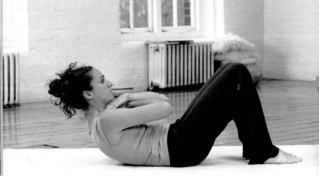

medium

- Lie flat on your back with your legs bent at 90°
- Place your hands across your chest, each touching the opposite shoulder

- Lift your head and shoulders towards your knees
- Lift your shoulders about 20cm off the floor and return slowly to the start position
Repeat 20 times

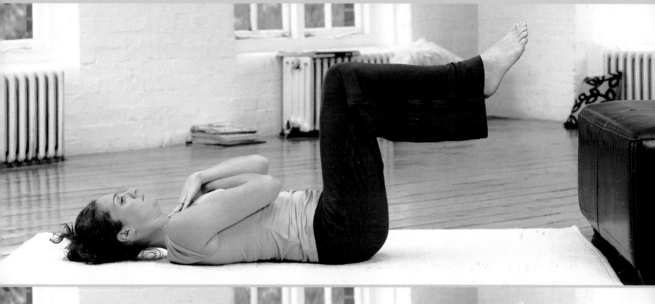

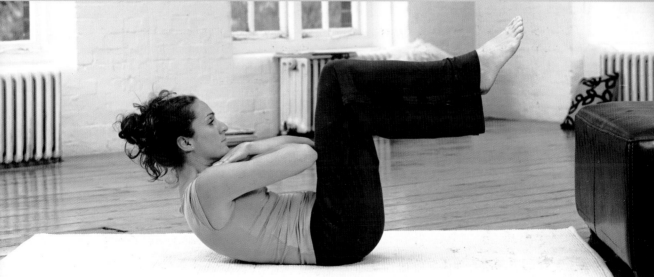

hard

• Lie flat on your back, bend your legs at 90°, then lift your legs in the air to make a 90° angle at the hip
• Place your hands across your chest, each touching the opposite shoulder

• Lift your head and shoulders towards your knees
• Touch your elbows on your knees and return slowly to the start position
Repeat 20 times

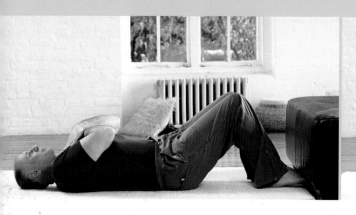 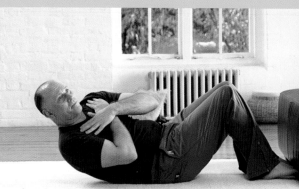

easy

• Lie flat on your back with your legs bent at 90°, then tuck your feet under a secure chair, table or door
• Place your hands across your chest, each touching the opposite shoulder

• Lift your head and shoulders towards your knees
• Point one elbow to the opposite knee, lifting your shoulders about 15cm off the floor
Return slowly to the start position and repeat 10 times on each side

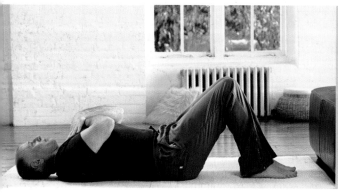 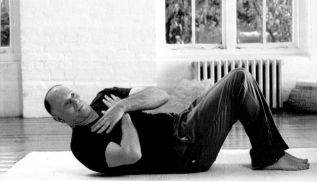

medium

• Lie flat on your back with your legs bent at 90° and place your hands across your chest, each touching the opposite shoulder
• Lift your head and shoulders towards your knees

• Point one elbow to the opposite knee, lifting your shoulders about 15cm off the floor
Return slowly to the start position and repeat 10 times on each side

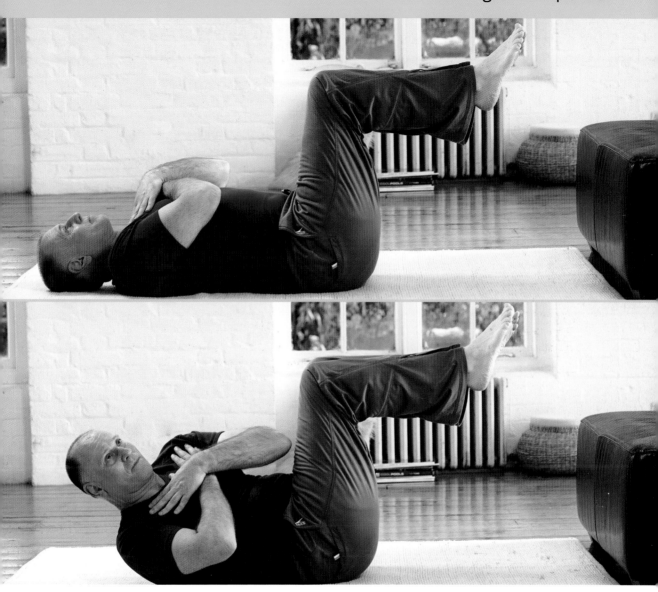

hard

• Lie flat on your back, bend your legs at 90°, then lift your legs in the air to make a 90° angle at the hip. Place your hands across your chest, each touching the opposite shoulder

• Lift your head and shoulders towards your knees
• Point one elbow to the opposite knee
Return slowly to the start position and repeat 10 times on each side

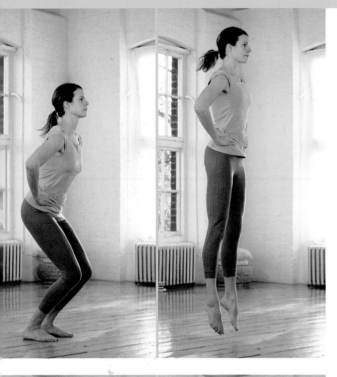

easy

• Stand upright with your feet shoulder-width apart and looking forwards
• Squat down about 45° and jump vertically upwards as high as you can
• Return to the start position before repeating
Repeat 20 times

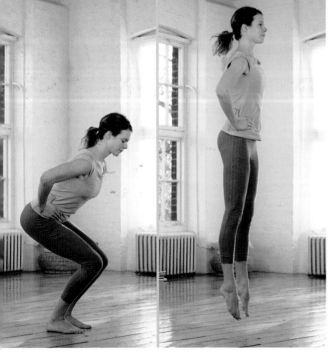

medium

• Stand upright with your feet shoulder-width apart and looking forwards
• Squat down about 90° and jump vertically upwards as high as you can
Repeat 20 times continuously without resting between

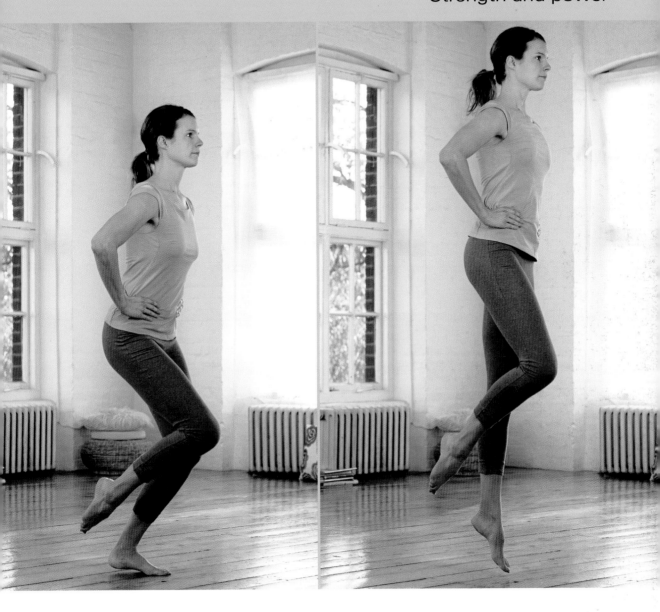

hard

• Stand upright with your feet shoulder-width apart and looking forwards
• On one leg, squat down as low as you can and jump vertically upwards as high as you can

Repeat 10 times
• Repeat with the other leg

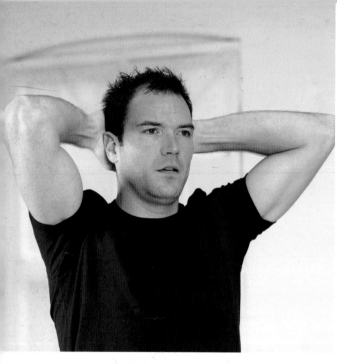

easy

• Stand upright, look forwards, interlock your fingers and place your hands behind your head
• Gently push your head backwards against your hands while pulling your hands forwards
• Hold for 10 seconds
Relax and repeat 5 times

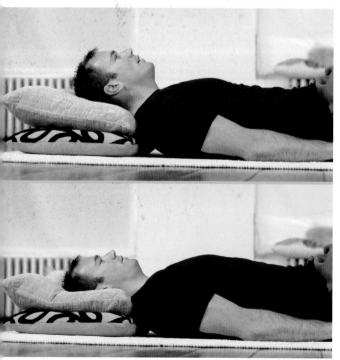

medium

• Lie on your back and place a cushion under the back of your head
• Push your head backwards against the cushion
• Hold for 10 seconds
Relax and repeat 5 times

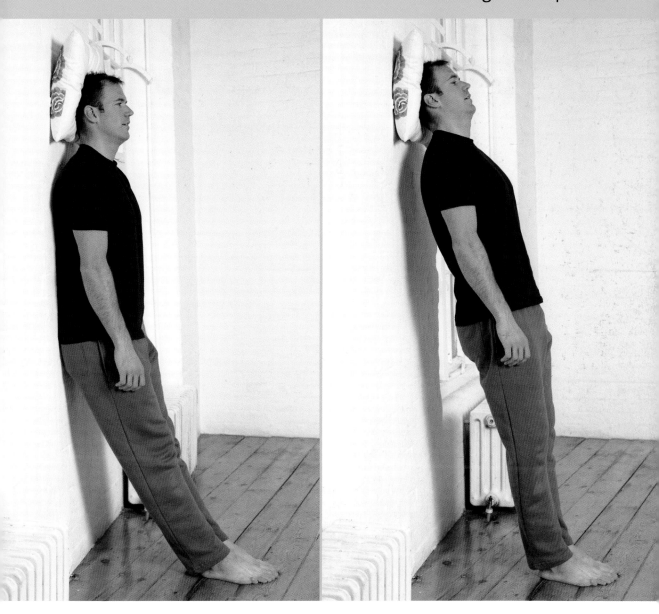

hard

• Stand with your back to a wall and take a small step away from the wall
• Lean back with your head and shoulders against a cushion resting on the wall

• Push your head backwards while lifting your shoulders away from the wall
Return to the start position and repeat 20 times

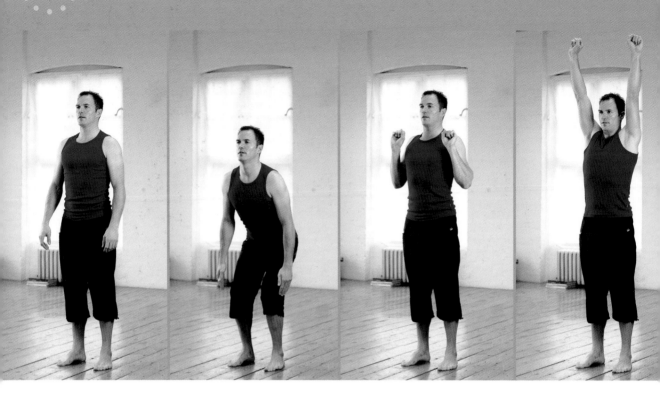

easy

- Stand with feet shoulder-width apart and arms by your side
- Keeping your back straight and looking forwards, bend the legs to 90°
- Straighten the legs and bend the arms, raising the hands to the front of your shoulders with the elbows down

- Extend the arms above your head until they are straight
- Return to the start position
Repeat 20 times

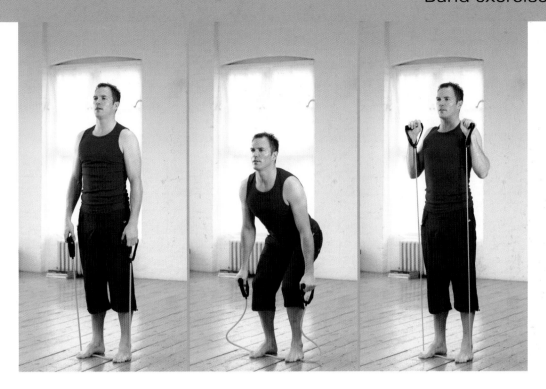

medium

- Place the middle of the band under your feet and hold a handle firmly in each hand
- Stand with feet shoulder-width apart and hands by your sides, holding the handles
- Keeping your back straight and, looking forwards, bend the legs to 90°

- Straighten the legs and bend the arms, raising the hands to the front of your shoulders with the elbows down
- Return to the start position
Repeat 20 times

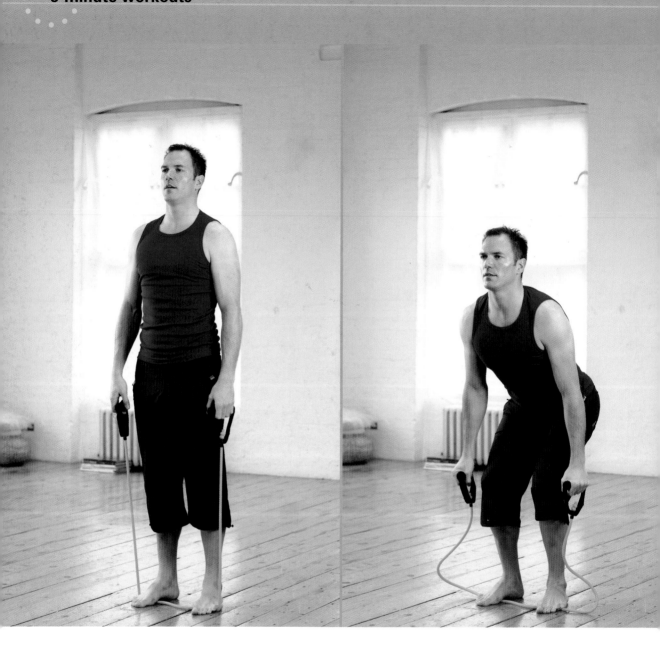

hard

- Place the middle of the band under your feet and hold a handle firmly in each hand
- Stand with feet shoulder-width apart and

hands by your sides, holding the handles
- Keeping your back straight and looking forwards, bend the legs to 90°

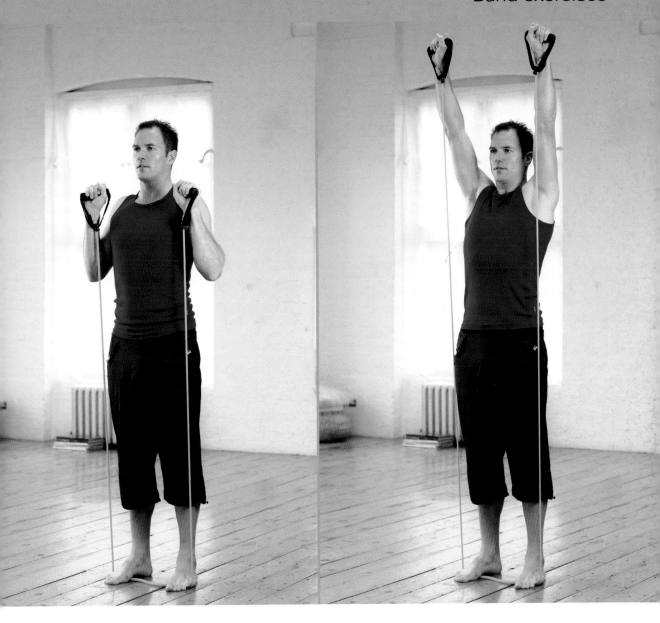

• Straighten the legs and bend the arms, raising the hands to the front of your shoulders with the elbows down

• Extend the arms above your head until they are straight
• Return to the start position
Repeat 20 times

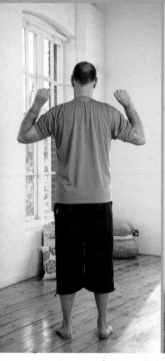
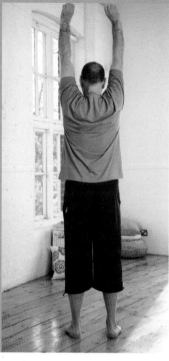

easy

• Stand with feet shoulder-width apart and arms bent with clenched hands level with your shoulders and elbows down
• Extend both arms upwards above your head until they are straight
• Return to the start position
Repeat 20 times

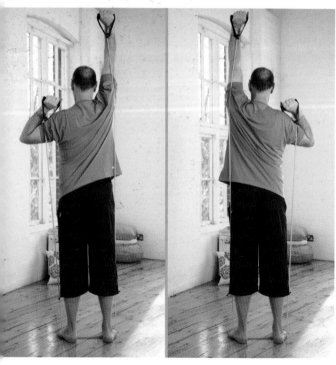

medium

• Place the middle of the band under your feet and hold a handle firmly in each hand
• Stand with feet shoulder-width apart and extend one arm upwards above your head until it is straight, keeping the other arm bent
• Return to the start position
• Change arms and repeat the above
Repeat 10 times

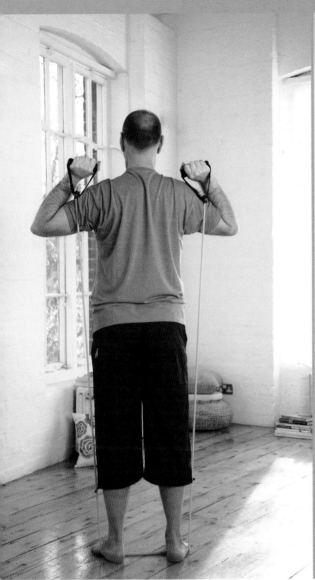
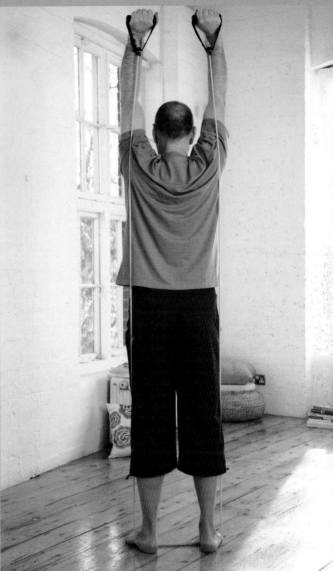

hard

- Place the middle of the band under your feet and hold a handle firmly in each hand
- Stand with feet shoulder-width apart and arms bent with hands level with your shoulders and elbows down

- Extend both arms upwards above your head until they are straight
- Return to the start position
Repeat 20 times

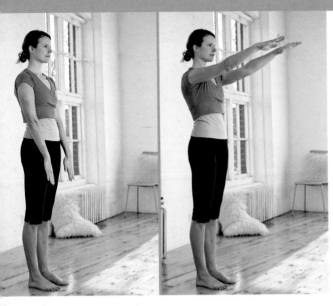

easy

- Stand with feet shoulder-width apart and hands by your thighs
- Keep the back straight and look forwards
- Keep the arms straight and raise both arms directly in front of you until your hands are level with the top of your head
- Return to start position

Repeat 20 times

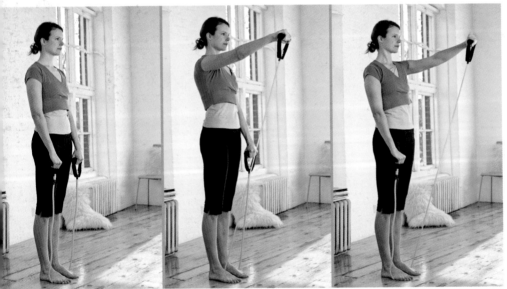

medium

- Place the middle of the band under your feet and hold a handle firmly in each hand
- Stand with feet shoulder-width apart and hands by your thighs, back straight

- Keep the arms straight and raise one arm directly in front of you until your hand is above your head. Return to start position

Repeat 10 times on each arm

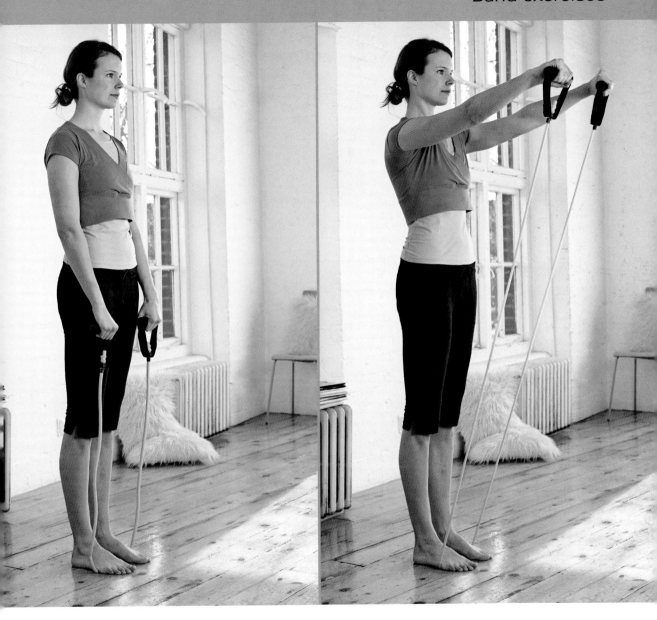

hard

- Stand with feet shoulder-width apart. Place the middle of the band under your feet and hold a handle firmly in each hand
- Keep the back straight and look forwards

- Keep the arms straight and raise both arms in front of you until your hands are level with the top of your head. Return to start position
Repeat 20 times

5-minute workouts   119

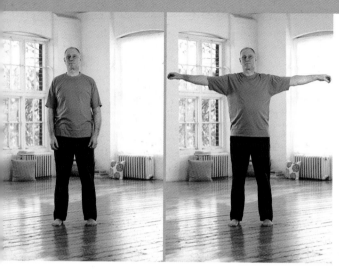

easy

• Stand with feet shoulder-width apart and palms resting on the sides of your thighs
• Keep the back straight and look forwards
• Keep the arms straight and raise both arms out to the sides until they reach shoulder level
• Return to the start position
Repeat 20 times

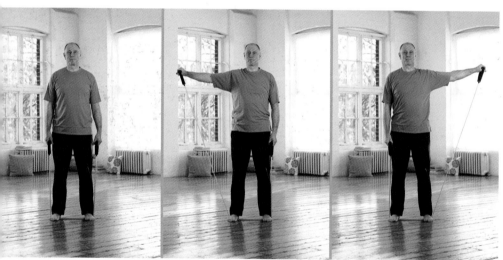

medium

• Place the middle of the band under your feet and hold a handle firmly in each hand
• Stand with feet shoulder-width apart and hands by the sides of your thighs
• Keep the back straight and look forwards

• Keep the arms straight and raise one arm out to the side until it reaches shoulder level
• Return to the start position
• Repeat with the other arm
Repeat 10 times

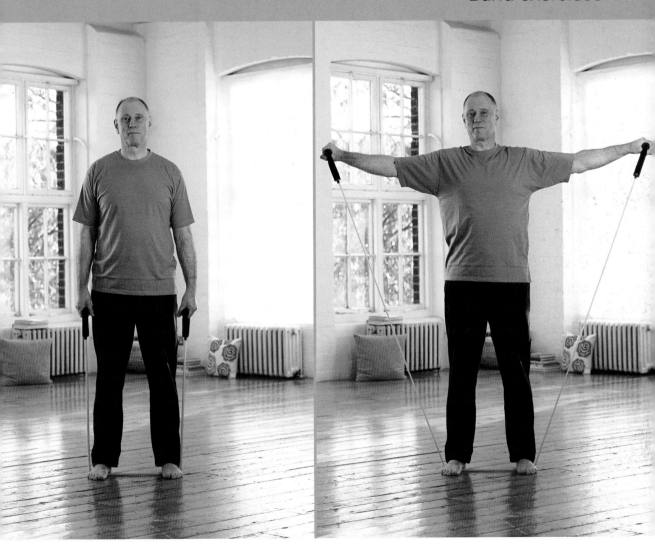

hard

- Place the middle of the band under your feet and hold a handle firmly in each hand
- Stand with feet shoulder-width apart and hands by the sides of your thighs
- Keep the back straight and look forwards

- Keep the arms straight and raise both arms out to the sides until they reach shoulder level
- Return to the start position
Repeat 20 times

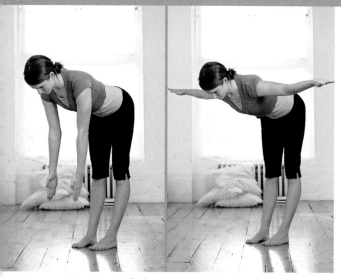

easy

• Stand with feet shoulder-width apart and bend forwards from the hips at an angle of just less than 90°, keeping your back straight
• Extend the arms in front of you so that they are pointing at the floor in front of you
• Keep the arms straight and lift them directly upwards to the sides of the body until they are level with your shoulders
• Return to the start position
Repeat 20 times

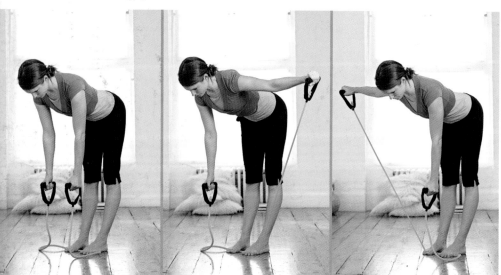

medium

• Place the middle of the band under your feet and hold a handle firmly in each hand
• Stand with feet shoulder-width apart and bend forwards from the hips at an angle of just less than 90°, keeping your back straight. Extend your arms towards the floor

• Raise one arm to the side of the body until the hand is level with your shoulders
• Return to the start position and repeat with the other arm
Repeat 20 times

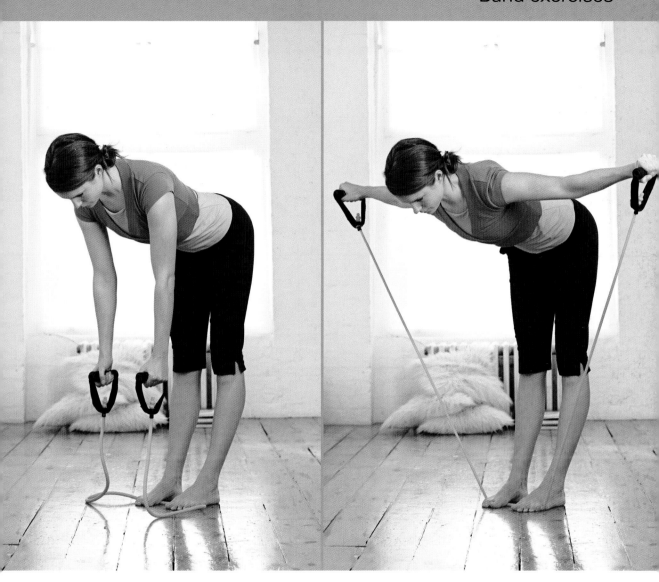

hard

- Place the middle of the band under your feet and hold a handle firmly in each hand
- Stand with feet shoulder-width apart and bend forwards from the hips at an angle of just less than 90°, keeping your back straight
- Extend the arms in front of you so that they

are pointing at the floor in front of you
- Keep the arms straight and lift them directly upwards to the sides of the body until they are level with your shoulders
- Return to the start position
Repeat 20 times

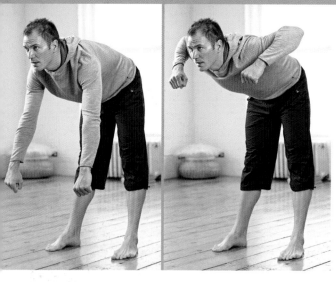

easy

• Stand with feet shoulder-width apart and bend forwards from the hips at an angle of just less than 90°, keeping your back straight
• Extend the arms in front of you so that they are pointing at the floor in front of you
• Bend the arms and bring your hands upwards until they touch your shoulders
• Return to the start position
Repeat 20 times

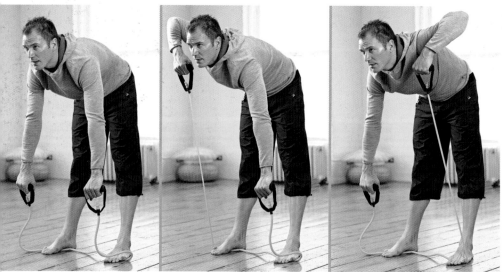

medium

• Place the middle of the band under your feet and hold a handle firmly in each hand
• Stand with feet shoulder-width apart and bend forwards from the hips at an angle of just less than 90°, keeping your back straight
• Extend the arms in front of you so that they

are pointing at the floor in front of you
• Bend one arm and bring your hand upwards until that hand touches your shoulder
• Return to the start position
• Repeat with the other arm
Repeat 10 times

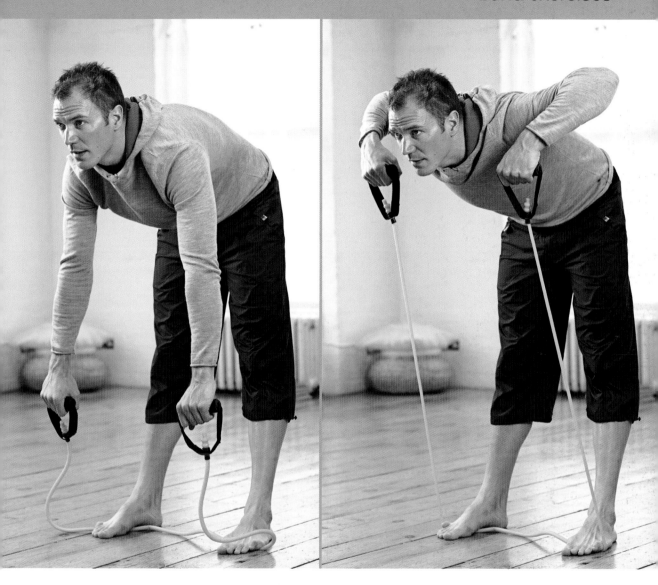

hard

• Place the middle of the band under your feet and hold a handle firmly in each hand
• Stand with feet shoulder-width apart and bend forwards from the hips at an angle of just less than 90°, keeping your back straight

• Extend the arms in front of you so that they are pointing at the floor in front of you
• Bending both arms, bring your hands upwards until they touch your shoulders
• Return to the start position
Repeat 20 times

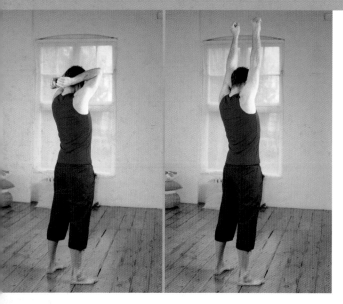

easy

• Stand upright with feet shoulder-width apart and looking forwards
• Extend the arms above your head and, keeping the elbows high, bend the arms until the hands are just above the shoulders
• Extend both arms above your head until they are straight
• Return to the start position
Repeat 20 times

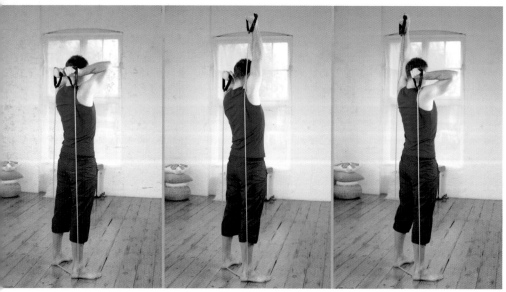

medium

• Place the middle of the band under your feet and hold a handle in each hand.
• Extend the arms above your head and keeping the elbows high, bend the arms until the hands are just above the shoulders
• Extend one arm above your head until straight
• Return to the start position
Repeat 10 times on each arm

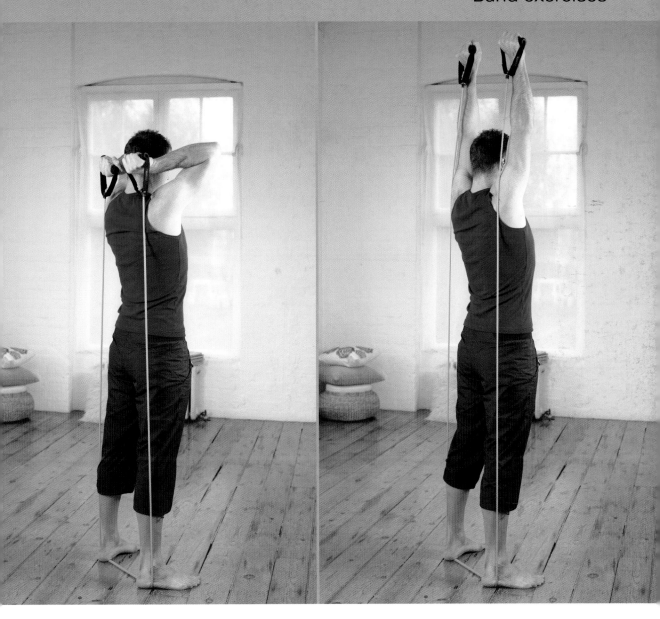

hard

- Place the middle of the band under your feet and hold a handle firmly in each hand
- Extend the arms above your head. Keeping the elbows high, bend the arms until the hands are just above the shoulders
- Extend both arms above your head until they are straight. Return to the start position
Repeat 20 times

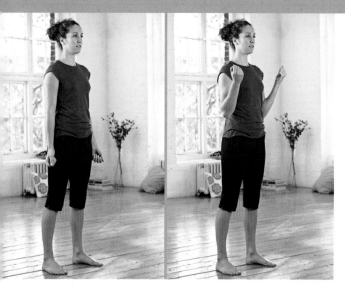

easy

• Stand with feet shoulder-width apart and arms by your sides, hands clenched
• Bend both arms to bring the hands towards your shoulder, keeping your elbows against your sides
• Return to the start position
Repeat 20 times

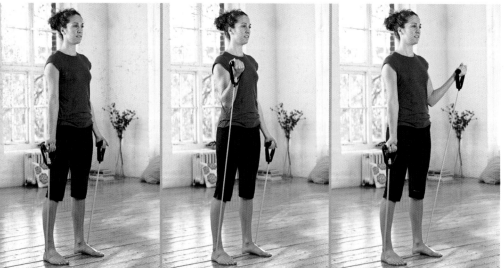

medium

• Place the middle of the band under your feet and hold a handle firmly in each hand
• Stand with feet shoulder-width apart and hands by your sides, palms facing forwards

• Bend one arm to bring the hand towards your shoulder, keeping your elbow tucked in
• Return to the start position
• Repeat with the other arm
Repeat 10 times on each arm

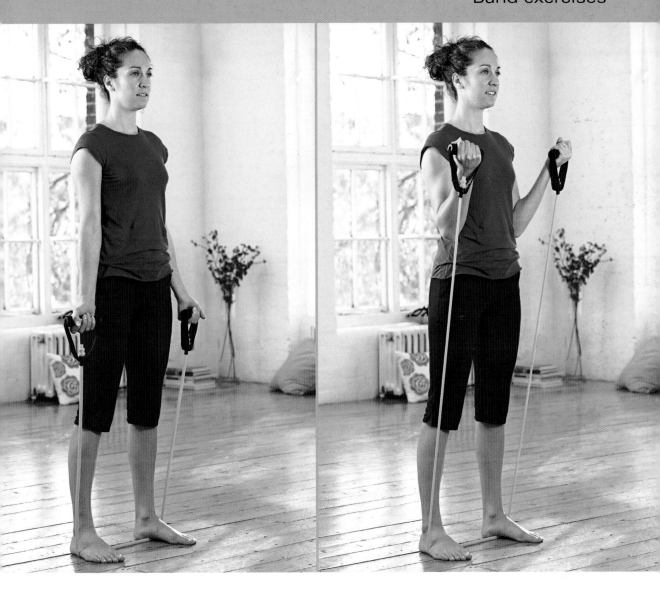

hard

• Place the middle of the band under your feet and hold a handle firmly in each hand
• Stand with feet shoulder-width apart and hands by your sides, palms facing forwards

• Bend both arms to bring the hands to your shoulders, keeping your elbows tucked in
• Return to the start position
Repeat 20 times

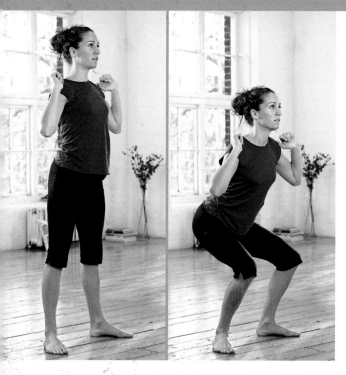

easy

• Stand with feet shoulder-width apart, arms bent with hands touching the shoulders, palms facing forwards and elbows touching your sides
• Keep your back straight and looking forwards, bend the legs to 90°
• Return to the start position
Repeat 20 times

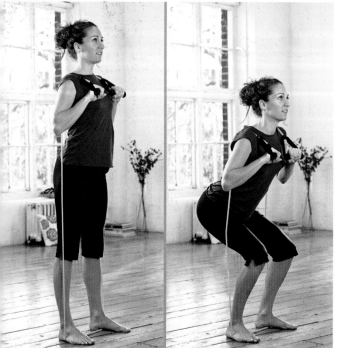

medium

• Place the middle of the band under your feet and, holding a handle firmly in each hand, pull the band over your shoulders
• Stand with feet shoulder-width apart, arms bent with hands touching the shoulders, palms facing forwards and elbows touching your sides
• Keep your back straight and, looking forwards, bend the legs to 90°
• Return to the start position
Repeat 20 times

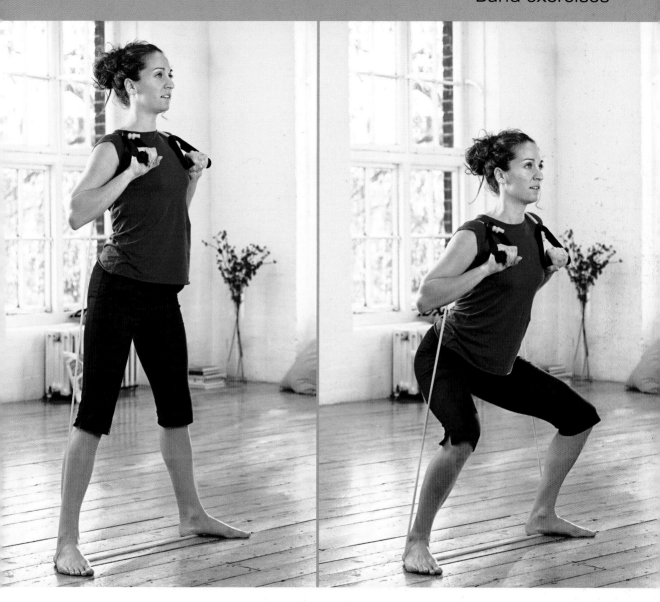

hard

• Place the middle of the band under your feet and, holding a handle firmly in each hand, pull the band over your shoulders. Stand with feet wide apart and pointing outwards
• Bend the arms with the hands touching the shoulders, palms facing forwards and elbows in
• Keep your back straight and, looking forwards, bend the legs to 90°
• Return to the start position
Repeat 20 times

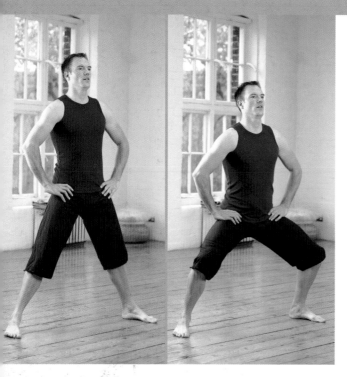

easy

• Stand with the legs wide apart and feet turned out with hands on hips
• Squat down, keeping your back straight and looking forwards
• Return to the start position
Repeat 20 times

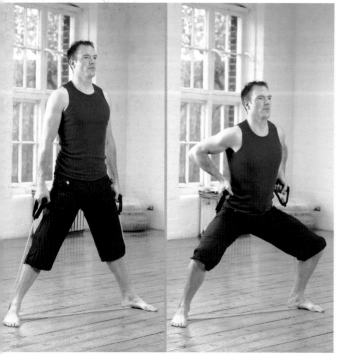

medium

• With the legs wide apart and feet turned out, stand on the middle of the band, holding the handles firmly
• Squat down, keeping your back straight and looking forwards
• Return to the start position
Repeat 20 times

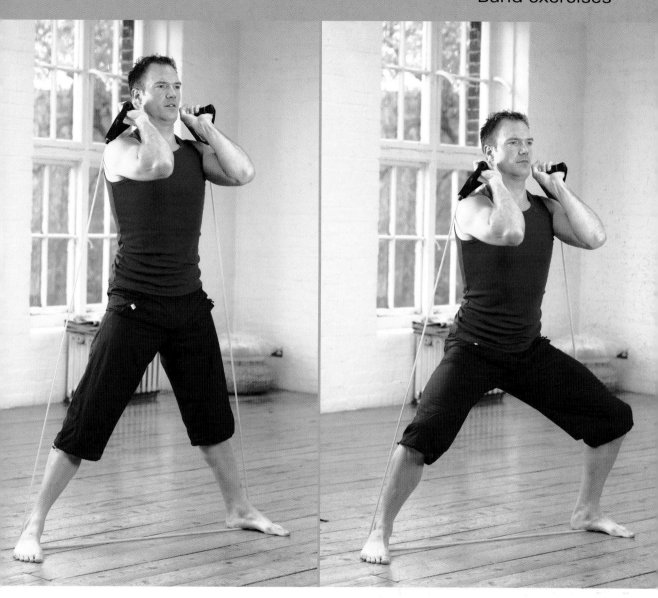

hard

- With the legs wide apart and feet turned out, stand on the middle of the band
- Hold the handles firmly and pull them over your shoulders

- Squat down, keeping your back straight and looking forwards
- Return to the start position
Repeat 20 times

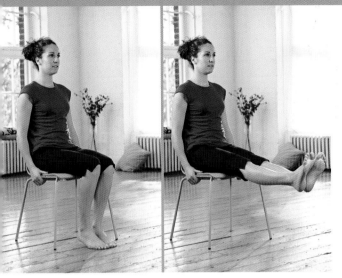

easy

• Sit upright, looking forwards, and hold the sides of the chair firmly
• Extend the legs straight in front of you, forming a straight line from hips to knees to ankles
• Return to the start position
Repeat 20 times

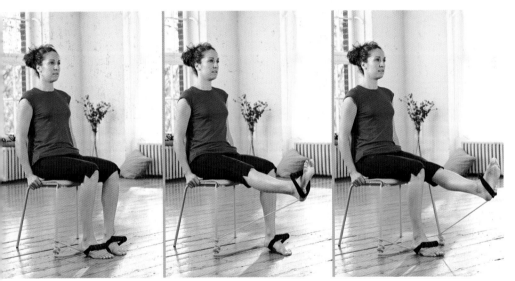

medium

• Place the band behind the front legs of the chair, looping the band around the legs
• Sit upright, looking forwards, and hold the sides of the chair firmly
• Place a foot through each of the handles
• Extend one leg straight in front of you, forming a straight line from hip to knee to ankle
• Return to the start position
• Repeat with the other leg
Repeat 20 times

134 GET FIT not fat

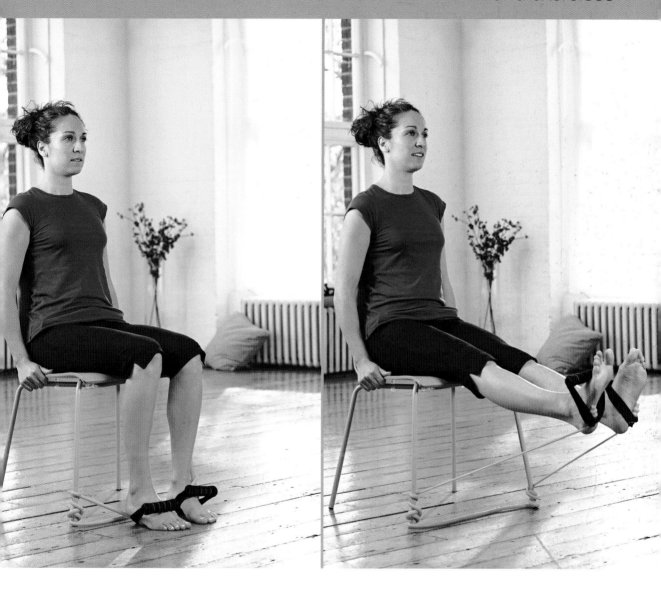

hard

- Place the band behind the front legs of the chair, looping the band around the legs
- Sit upright, looking forwards, and hold the sides of the chair firmly
- Place a foot through each of the handles
- Extend both legs straight in front of you,

forming a straight line from hips to knees to ankles
- Return to the start position
Repeat 20 times

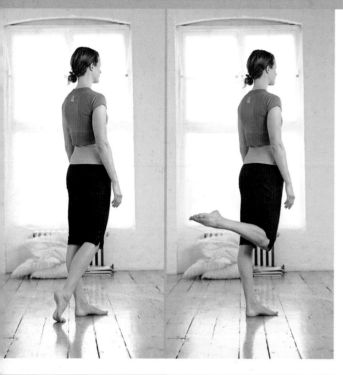

easy

• Stand upright with feet shoulder-width apart and looking forwards
• Hold a chair or the wall to stabilise the body if required
• Lift the lower part of one leg behind you as high as possible, aiming to touch the heel of the foot on your bum
• Return to the start position
• Repeat with the other leg
Repeat 10 times

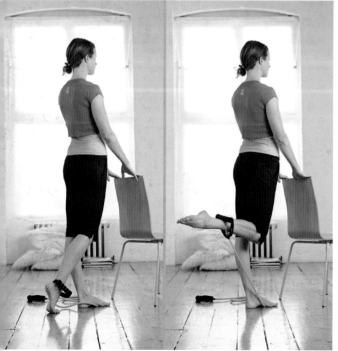

medium

• Place one foot through the handle and stand on the band, adjusting the tension to create a medium resistance
• Stand upright with feet shoulder-width apart and looking forwards
• Hold a chair or the wall to stabilise the body
• Lift the lower part of one leg behind you as high as possible, aiming to touch the heel of the foot on your bum
• Return to the start position
Repeat 10 times
• Repeat with the other leg

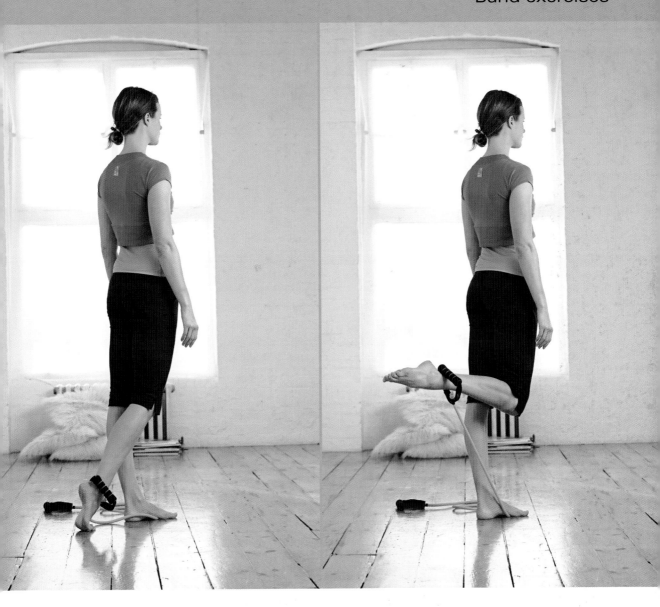

hard

• Place one foot through the handle and stand on the band, adjusting the tension to create a hard resistance
• Stand upright and looking forwards
• Lift the lower part of one leg behind you as high as possible, aiming to touch the heel of the foot on your bum
• Return to the start position
Repeat 10 times
• Repeat with the other leg

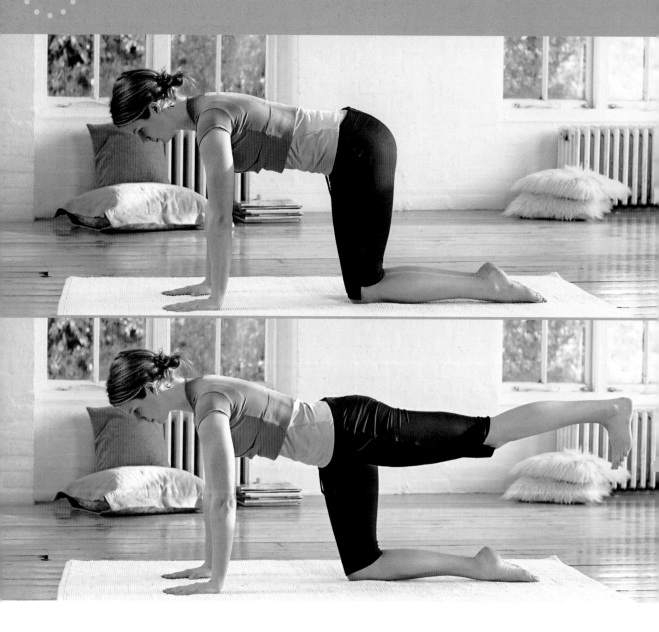

easy

• Start on all fours with your weight evenly distributed and looking forwards
• Extend one leg straight behind you, making a straight line between shoulder, hip, knee and ankle

• Return to the start position
• Repeat with the other leg
Repeat 10 times

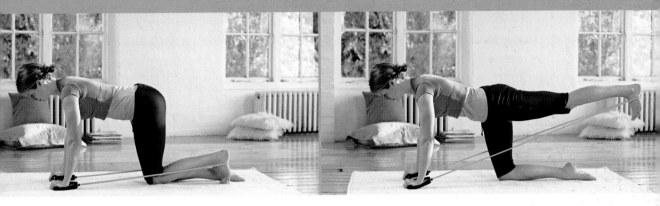

medium

- Start on all fours with your weight evenly distributed and looking forwards
- Hold the handles of the band firmly in each hand and place the middle of the band on the sole of one foot

- Extend the leg straight behind you, making a straight line between your shoulder, hip, knee and ankle
- Return to the start position
- Repeat with the other leg
Repeat 10 times

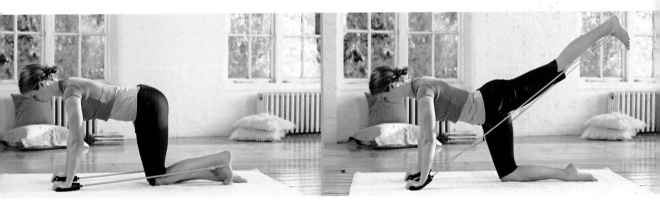

hard

- Start on all fours with your weight evenly distributed and looking forwards
- Hold the handles of the band firmly in each hand and place the middle of the band on the sole of one foot

- Extend the leg straight behind you and lift up as high as possible without turning out the hip
- Return to the start position
- Repeat with the other leg
Repeat 10 times

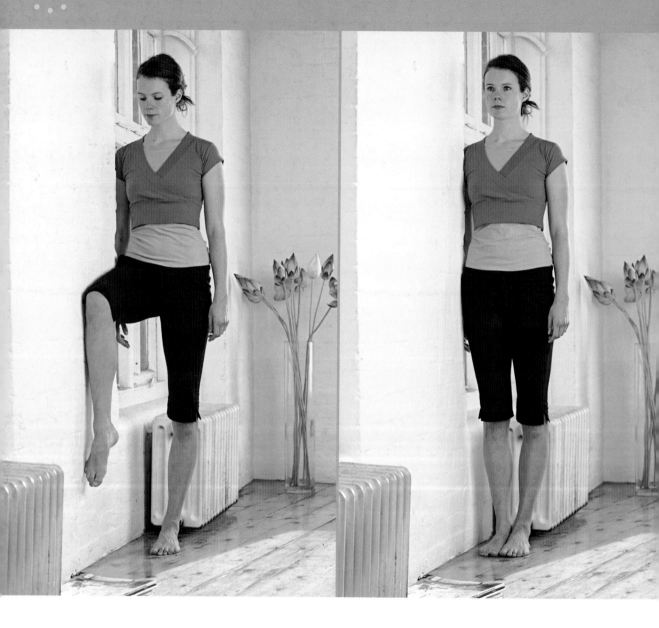

easy

• Stand side on next to a wall, lift the knee closest to the wall so that the thigh is parallel to the floor and place the knee and lower leg against the wall

• Push the knee and lower leg against the wall
• Hold for 10 seconds
• Return the foot to the floor
• Turn the body and repeat with the other leg
Repeat 4 times

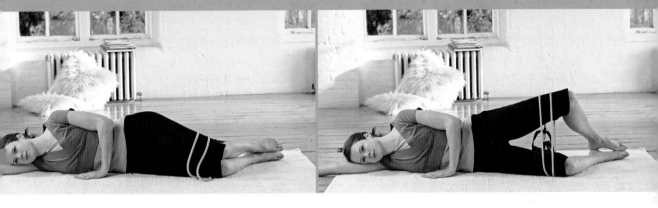

medium

- Wrap the band securely around your knees, leaving it loose enough to require a moderate contraction to lift the knee
- Lie on your side with your lower arm extended above your head and the upper arm supporting your body

- Keep the legs together, bent at 45° and making a straight line from shoulders to hips to feet
- Keeping the feet together lift the upper knee as high as possible
- Return to the start position
Repeat 20 times on each leg

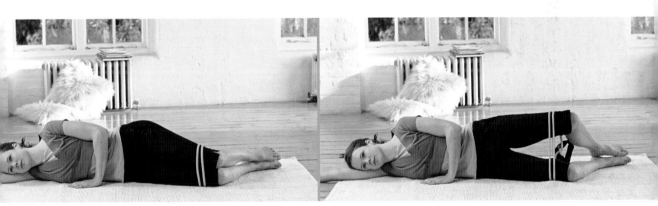

hard

- Wrap the band securely around your knees, so it requires a hard contraction to lift the knee
- Lie on your side with your lower arm extended above your head and the upper arm supporting your body

- Keep the legs together, bent at 45°
- Keeping the feet together, lift the upper knee as high as possible
- Return to the start position
Repeat 20 times on each leg

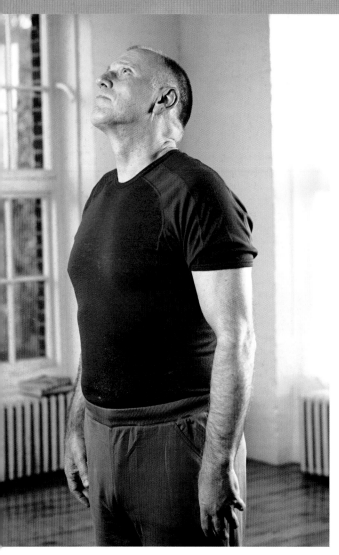

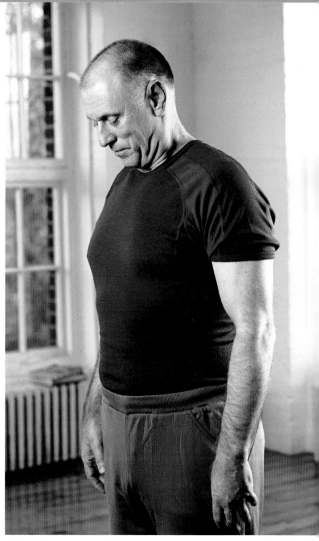

Neck extension

- Keep your body upright and stable
- Raise your chin as high as possible without leaning backwards, keeping your mouth closed
- Hold for 20–30 seconds

Neck flexion

- Keep your body upright and stable
- Lower your chin to your chest without leaning forwards
- Hold for 20–30 seconds

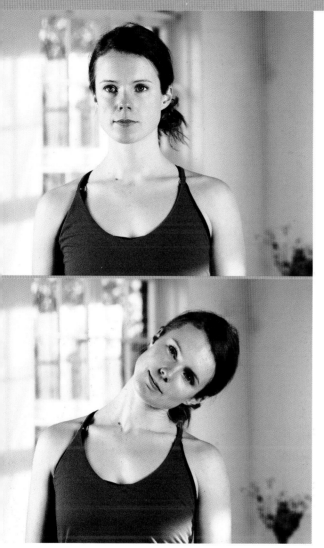

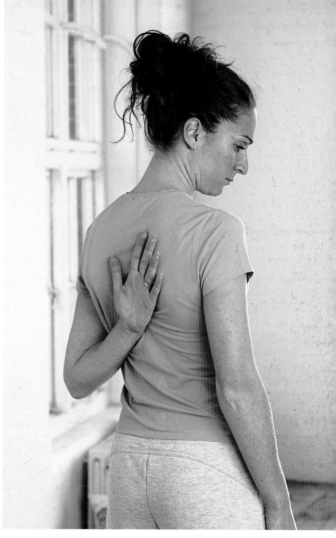

Side neck

• Keep your body upright and stable
• Lower your ear towards the shoulder on the same side
• When you feel a stretch hold for 20–30 seconds
Repeat on the other side

Neck stretch

• Keep your body upright and stable. Place your left hand behind your back as high up the back as possible
• Look downwards to your right side
• When you feel the stretch hold for 20–30 seconds
Repeat on the other side

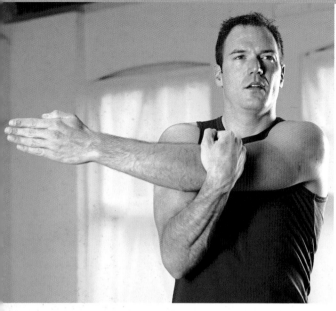

Back of shoulder

• Stand upright with feet shoulder-width apart and looking forwards
• Bring one arm across your chest towards the opposite shoulder without rotating the upper body
• Cup the elbow with your hand and pull the arm towards your chest until you feel a stretch in the back of your shoulder
• Hold for 20–30 seconds
Repeat with the other arm

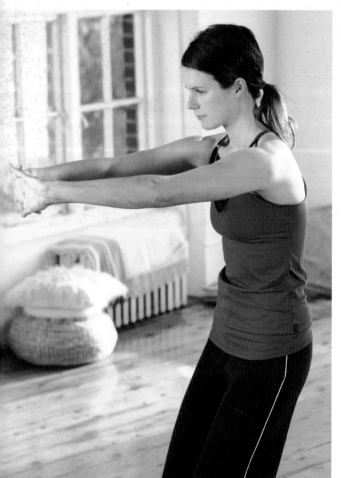

Upper back

• Stand upright with feet shoulder-width apart and looking forwards
• Interlock your fingers with palms facing outwards and stretch your arms out in front of you
• Round your shoulders and push out your shoulder blades
• Hold for 20–30 seconds

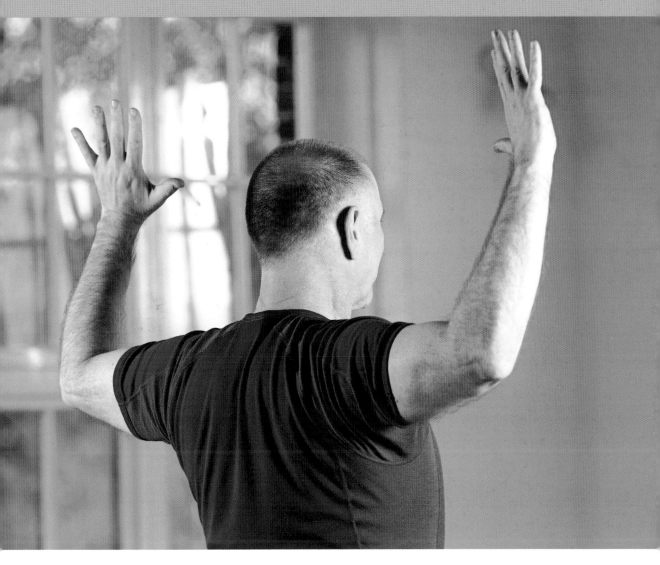

Chest

• Stand upright with feet shoulder-width apart and looking forwards
• Bend your arms at 90° and raise them out to the sides until your elbows are at shoulder height

• Pull your elbows backwards and push your chest out until you feel a stretch across your chest
• Hold for 20–30 seconds

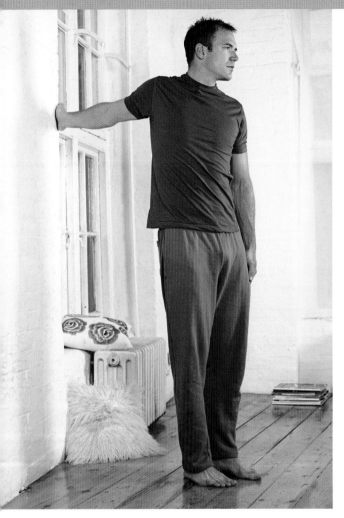

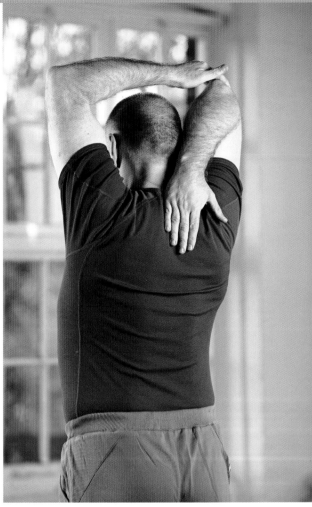

Biceps

• Stand upright next to a wall or door, looking forwards
• Place the palm of one hand against the wall at shoulder height
• Keeping the arm straight, turn the body away from the wall until you feel a stretch along the front of your arm
• Hold for 20–30 seconds
Repeat with the other arm

Triceps

• Stand upright with feet shoulder-width apart
• Lift one arm above your head and bend it at the elbow with the hand pointing down your back
• Cup the elbow with the opposite hand and ease the elbow towards your head until you feel a stretch in the back of the upper arm
• Hold for 20–30 seconds
Repeat with the other arm

Side stretch

• Standing upright and looking forwards,
extend both arms above your head
• Without bending forwards or backwards lean
to one side
• Hold for 20–30 seconds
• Return to the start position
Repeat for the other side

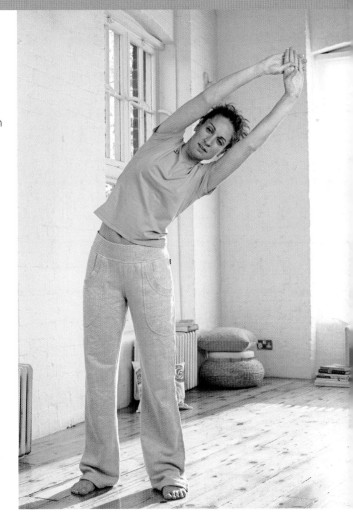

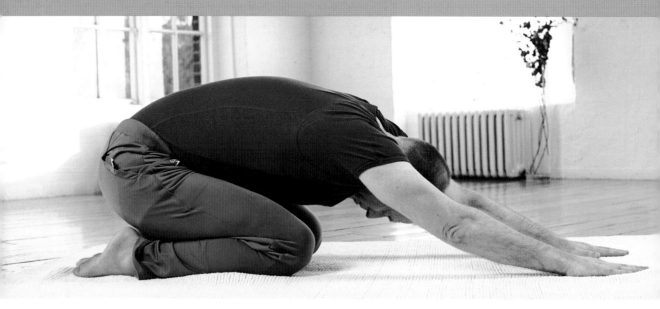

Lower back

- Kneel down on the floor and sit on your heels
- Curl your body over your thighs

- Place your forehead as close to the floor as possible, arms outstretched in front of you
- Relax and hold for 20–30 seconds

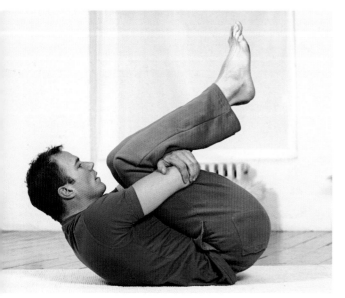

Back

- Lie on your back and curl your lower body up towards your head
- Place your arms behind your knees and pull your knees to your chest
- Tuck your head into your knees and relax
- Hold for 20–30 seconds

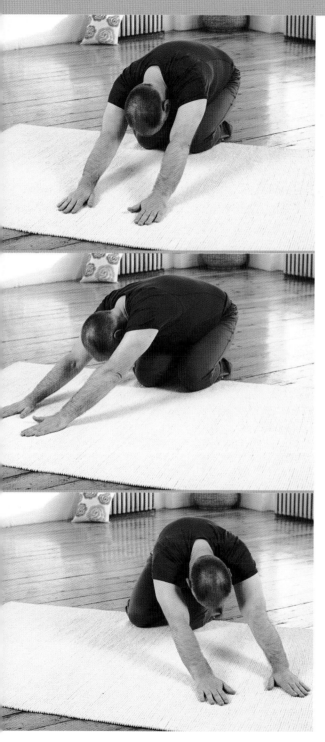

Upper body stretch

• Kneel down on the floor and sit on
your heels
• Curl your body over your thighs
• Place your forehead as close to the floor as
possible, arms outstretched in front of you
• Keeping your forehead near to the floor, walk
your hands slowly to the right until you feel a
stretch along your upper body
• Relax and hold for 20–30 seconds
• Walk your hands to the left, relax and hold
for 20–30 seconds

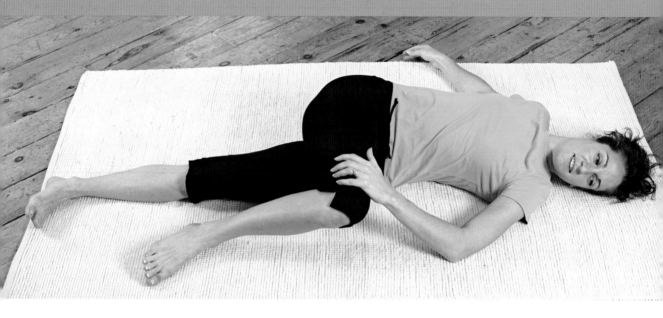

Lower back and hips

• Lie on your back and bring your right knee towards your chest
• Place your left hand on your right knee
• Keeping your shoulders on the floor, ease the right leg across your body until you feel a stretch across your hip and lower back
• Hold for 20–30 seconds
Repeat with the left leg

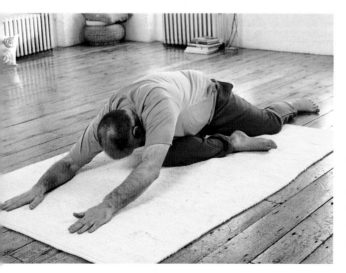

Hips – Z-stretch

• Kneel on the floor, then extend one leg directly backwards
• Keeping your legs in place, roll the hip out to sit on the floor
• Curl your body over your front leg
• Aim your forehead towards the floor and extend your arms in front of you
• Relax and hold for 20–30 seconds

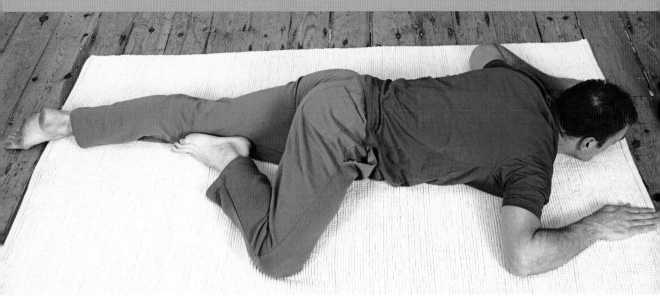

Hip

- Lie face down with legs extended
- Bend one knee, placing the sole of the foot on your thigh
- Relax and hold for 20–30 seconds
Repeat with the other leg

Hip – standing

- Standing upright and looking forwards, cross your right foot over your left
- Without bending forwards or backwards, lean to the left side and extend your right arm above your head
- Hold for 20–30 seconds
- Return to the start position
Repeat with the left leg and left arm

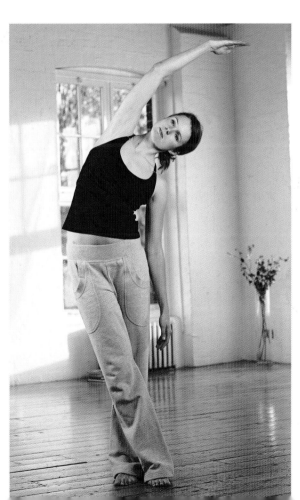

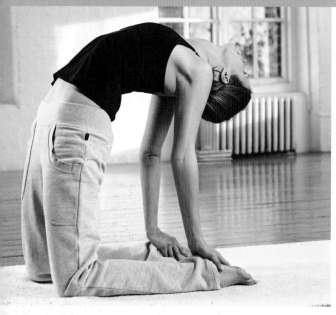

Camel

• Kneel on the floor and place your hands on your heels
• Starting from your knees and keeping your arms extended, slowly roll your body back, pushing out your tummy, then your chest, and looking backwards
• Hold for 20–30 seconds

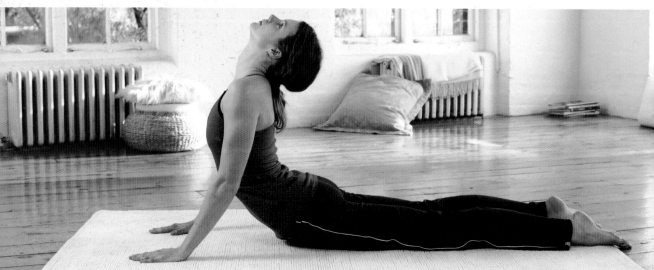

Back raise

• Lie face down with your arms bent to the sides and your hands next to your shoulders

• Keeping your hips on the floor, extend your arms and lift your upper body upwards and look to the ceiling
• Hold for 20–30 seconds

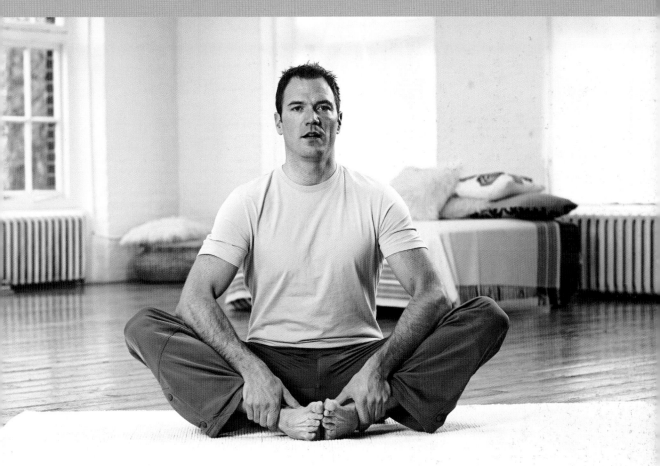

Groin

- Sit up straight on the floor and place the soles of the feet together
- Hold the feet with both hands and place your elbows on your knees

- Press your knees towards the floor until you feel a stretch
- Hold for 20–30 seconds

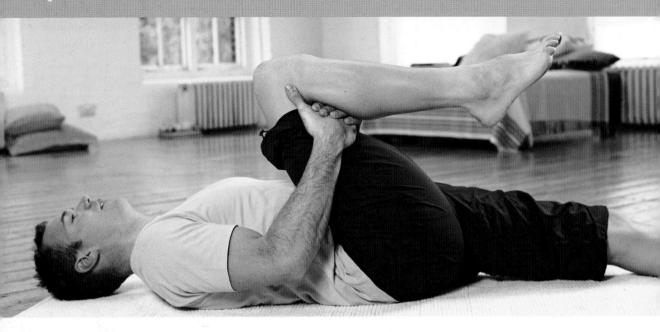

Bum

• Lie on your back on the floor
• Leave one leg straight and, keeping your shoulders on the floor, bend the knee of your other leg and bring it towards your chest

• Place both hands behind the bent knee and pull the knee towards your chest
• Hold for 20–30 seconds
Repeat with the other leg

Bum and hip

• Lie on your back on the floor with both legs bent
• Place the ankle of one leg on the knee of the other leg
• Place both hands behind the bent knee and pull the knee towards your chest
• Hold for 20–30 seconds
Repeat with the other leg

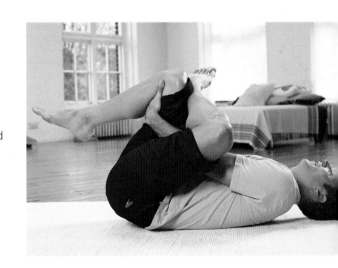

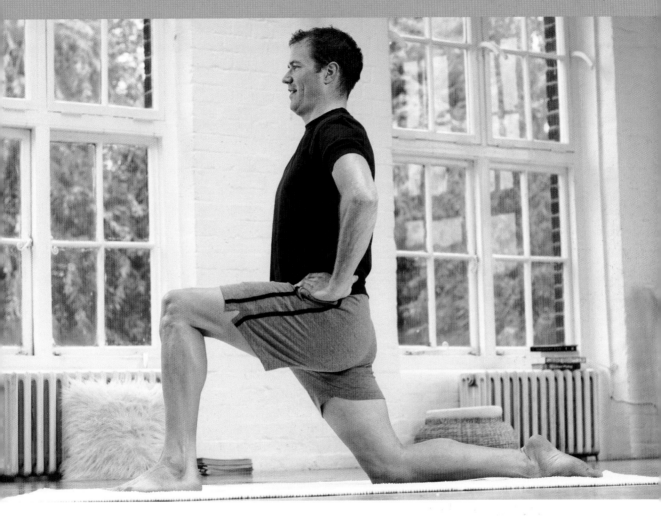

Hip flexor

- In the lunge position drop the back knee to the floor well behind the hip
- With the back knee on the floor and hands on hips, extend forwards so that the front knee is at 90°

- Feel the stretch on the front of the hip joint and the thigh
- Hold for 20–30 seconds
Repeat with the other leg

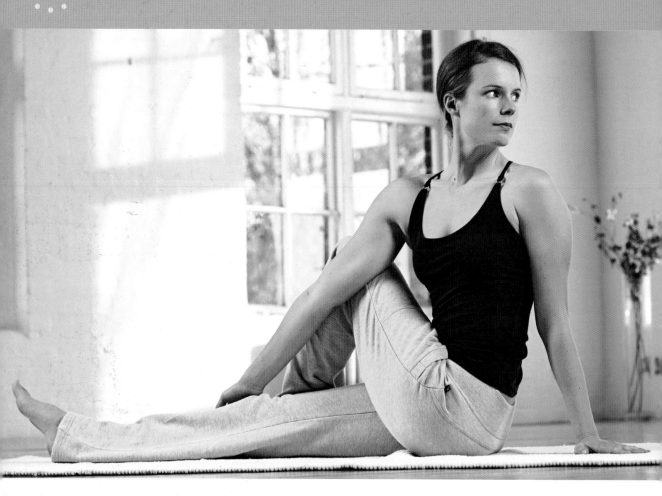

Seated outer thigh

- Sit on the floor with your legs straight in front
- Bend the left leg and place the foot over the right leg

- Rotate your body and extend your right arm and place it over the left leg
- Gently ease your left knee to the right
- Hold for 20–30 seconds
Repeat with the other leg

Hamstring – seated

• Sit on the floor, body upright, with one leg extended in front of you and the other leg bent with your foot in your groin
• Bend forwards, starting at the lower back and working up to your head, reaching for your toes until you feel a stretch along the back of your upper leg
• Hold for 20–30 seconds
Repeat with the other leg

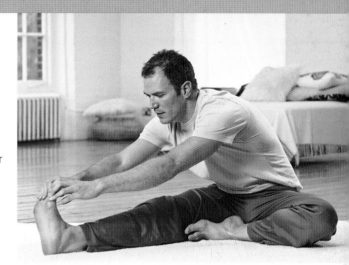

Hamstring – standing

• Stand upright with feet shoulder-width apart and looking forwards
• Take a step forwards
• Bend the back leg, keeping the front leg straight
• Bend forwards and pull the toes of the front leg towards you until you feel a stretch along the back of the upper leg
• Hold for 20–30 seconds
Repeat with the other leg

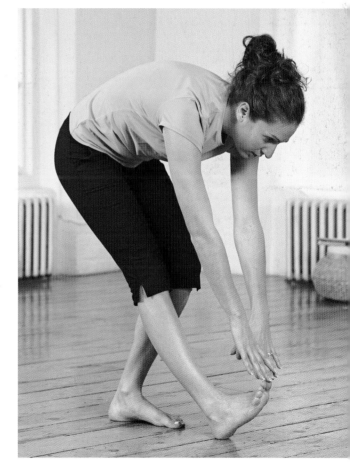

5-minute workouts 157

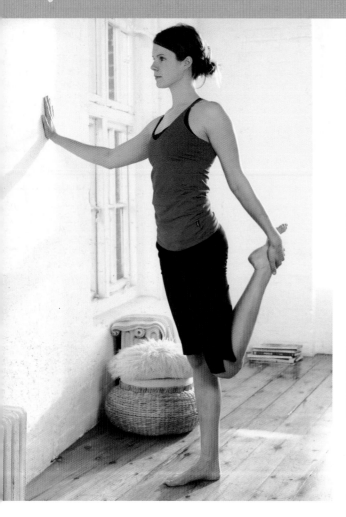

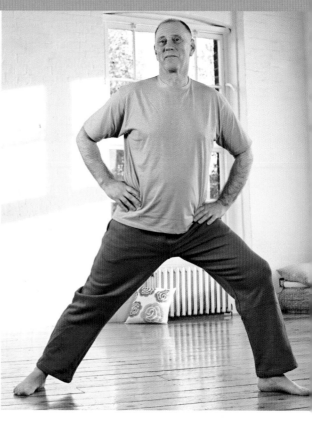

Inner thigh

• Stand with feet slightly more than shoulder-width apart
• Looking forwards, keep your body upright
• Keep one leg straight and bend the other leg until you feel a stretch in the inner thigh
• Hold for 20–30 seconds
Repeat with the other leg

Thigh

• Stand upright next to a wall
• Bend the knee of one leg and pull the heel towards your bum (hold onto the wall for stability if required)
• Hold the ankle of the bent leg and pull the foot into your bum without leaning forwards (keep a straight line between shoulder, hip and knee)
• Hold for 20–30 seconds
Repeat with the other leg

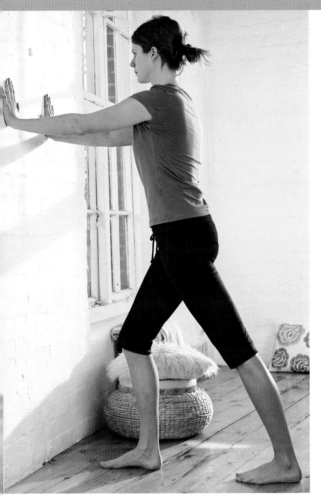

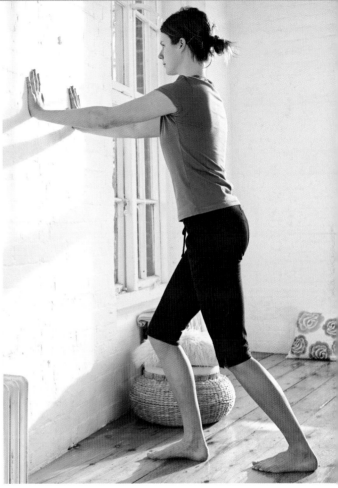

Upper calf

• Stand in a lunge position with the front foot about 30cm away from a wall or a chair
• Lean on the wall or chair and bend the leading leg until you feel a stretch in the calf of your straight leg
• Hold for 20–30 seconds
Repeat with the other calf

Lower calf

• Stand in a lunge position with the front foot about 30cm away from a wall or a chair
• Lean on the wall or chair
• With the leading leg bent, bend the back leg until you feel a stretch in the lower part of the calf
• Hold for 20–30 seconds
Repeat with the other calf

10-minute

workouts

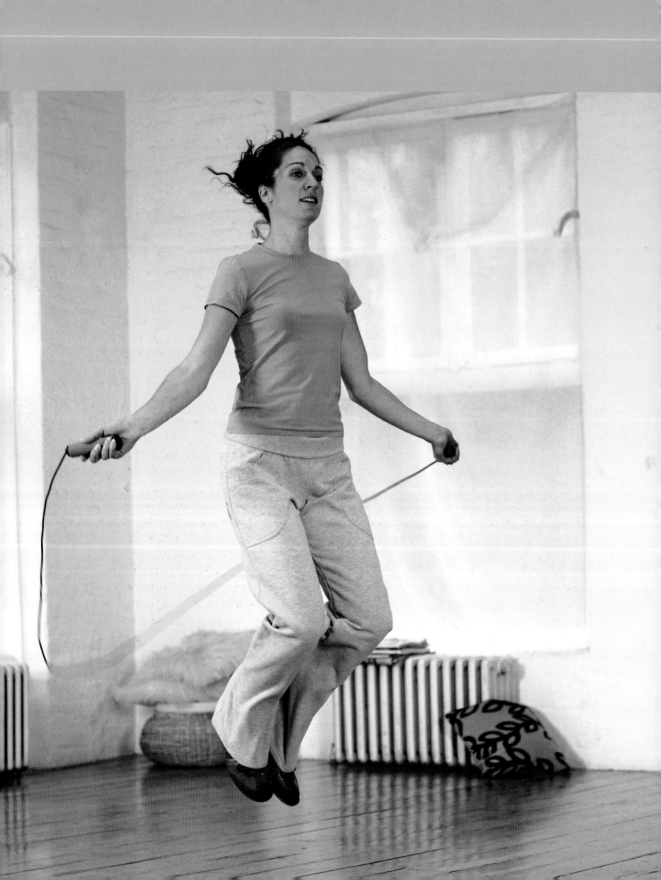

The 5-minute exercises can be enjoyed any time, anywhere and you can easily fit them into your day. Sometimes, however, you may have a little more time available. This chapter covers 10-minute workouts, and focuses on a variety of exercises that extract elements of the 5- and 30-minute workouts with the emphasis on strength endurance.

Strength endurance

Strength-endurance exercises focus on your ability to maintain strength exercises over time. This type of fitness is very important for all forms of exercise and daily living. Any repetitive activity that requires you to maintain the action for a short duration of time requires strength endurance. Routine activities that require strength endurance include hill walking, stair climbing, gardening and vacuum cleaning. Improving your strength (the ability to produce force on a single occasion) will lead to an improvement in your exercise capacity but the addition of strength-endurance training will significantly improve both exercise and the ease with which you perform daily living activities. Combining the 5-minute exercises in Chapter 5 with the strength-endurance exercises in this chapter will result in enhanced flexibility, strength and strength endurance – all of which will improve your quality of life, health and well-being.

Strength-endurance exercises tend to be at a higher intensity compared with 30-minute exercises that focus on cardio-respiratory (heart and lung) fitness and although the rating (easy, medium or hard) of the exercises you choose may be somewhat less than you would choose for a 5-minute exercise, repeating the exercise and combining exercises without recovery often makes 10-minute exercise more intense.

10-minute workout: upper-body strength circuit exercises

Strength and power:
- Push-up

Band exercises:
- Shoulder press • Tricep curl • Bicep curl
- Anterior deltoid • Medial deltoid
- Posterior deltoid

There is a number of different ways in which to improve your strength endurance, including circuits, stair climbing, skipping and hard-intensity exercise.

Circuits

Circuits encompass a number of specific exercises that target certain muscle groups and sometimes skills (such as skiing) associated with the goals of the session. For example, if you are targeting lower back strength you will want to select exercises that concentrate on back, stomach and core muscles. To stress muscular endurance optimally, the recovery periods between exercises are often relatively short to allow only partial recovery. During a 10-minute session you would normally select between six and ten exercises from the 5-minute exercises chapter and run through them until your 10 minutes are complete. There is a number of formats that you can use with circuits. You can select six to eight different exercises and run through them sequentially, or you can select only three exercises and sequentially run through the circuit, repeating each exercise three times. In addition to the 5-minute exercises you could incorporate stair climbing or skipping for short bursts (1–2 minutes) into your circuit to add variety.

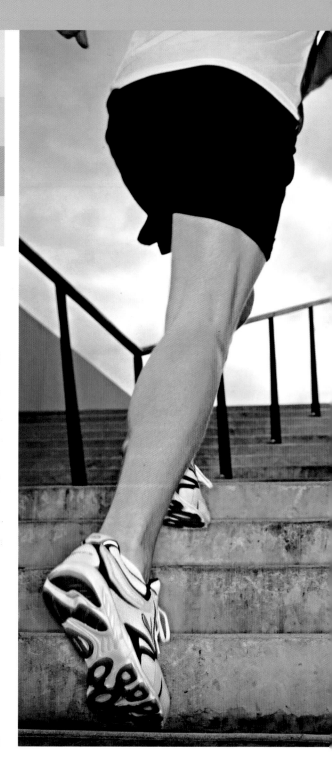

10-minute workout: lower-body strength circuit exercises

Strength and power:
• Squat • Jump squat

Band exercises:
• Leg extension • Leg curl

Skipping:
2 minutes

You can variously alter the intensity of circuits. Simply increasing the intensity of each exercise will lead to a progressive overload stimulus. Adding in other exercises and ensuring you complete them all within the 10-minute session will increase the speed and therefore the intensity of the circuit. Increasing the number of times you complete a small circuit will also increase intensity: for example, if you choose three exercises and are able to repeat each exercise twice in the first few weeks, aim to repeat each exercise three times after, say, three weeks.

Stair climbing

This is hard work! Climbing stairs slowly is often more intense than moderate or fast walking on the flat because a greater amount of energy is required. You don't need long flights – just enough stairs to make you work your muscles hard to get to the top. It is simple enough to increase the intensity of stair climbing: just climb faster. To help your motivation, keep a record of how many steps you can climb in 10 minutes and try to beat that number every time you stair climb.

Coming back down the stairs is good for you too! The increased loading on the legs as you descend increases muscular strength and

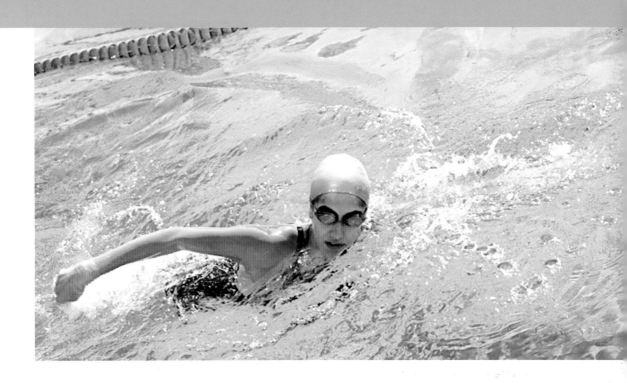

bone strength and is a great addition to your exercise programme.

You can also target strength endurance by walking, jogging, running and cycling uphill. So if you don't have a suitable flight of stairs find a hill close to home or work and get climbing!

Skipping

Skipping is a great exercise for strength endurance. The energy required makes it demanding and the increased load-bearing on the bones makes it an excellent exercise for bone health. You can increase the intensity by increasing the speed at which you skip. If you don't have a skipping rope, jumping on the spot, mimicking the action, is good enough!

Hard-intensity exercise

Taking any of the 30-minute exercises in Chapter 7 and increasing the intensity to hard will work strength endurance. Any

exercise that you find difficult to maintain for 10 minutes will stress your strength endurance. For example, rather than walking for 30 minutes, try running for 10 minutes. The increased load-bearing on the legs from running will lead to strength endurance of the lower body. If you already run for 30 minutes, increase the speed, and therefore the intensity, to build up strength endurance. On a bike you can focus on strength endurance by using a very difficult gear – this is similar to cycling uphill. In swimming you can choose a more difficult stroke to work strength endurance, or alternatively you can use floats between your legs and swim with your arm power only to work on upper-body strength endurance or hold the float and kick for lower-body strength endurance. Basically, strength-endurance exercise is hard work, but it doesn't last that long and, remember, nothing good comes easy!

30-minute

workouts

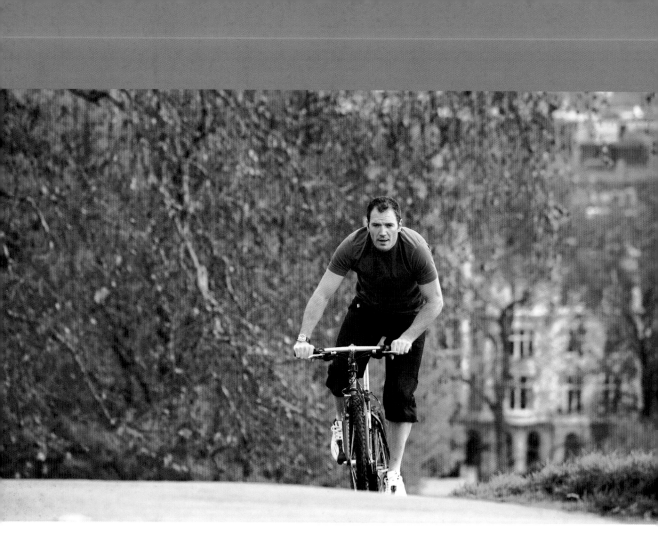

The recommended amount of exercise for optimal health and disease prevention is five 30-minute episodes of moderate-intensity exercise per week. While this may appear to be a simple message we need to clarify the sort of questions it usually raises, typically: what type of exercise does this include?; what does moderate intensity mean?; how will I know what intensity I am exercising at? In addition, one of the biggest problems with 30-minute exercise sessions is that they can be monotonous and boring. This chapter answers these questions and gives you ideas on how to make 30-minute sessions an enjoyable part of your weekly routine.

What type of exercise?

The answer is simple: any exercise that increases your physical activity and causes a rise in heart rate. That can be any form of activity from housework and gardening to football, walking, jogging, cycling and swimming. The key factor in choosing which type of exercise is to select those that fit into your daily routine and, importantly, to ensure they are activities you enjoy. Many of us use the excuse that we don't have time for 30 minutes of exercise, whereas more often the underlying problem is that we find 30 minutes of a single exercise dull and boring. To enhance the enjoyment of your workouts

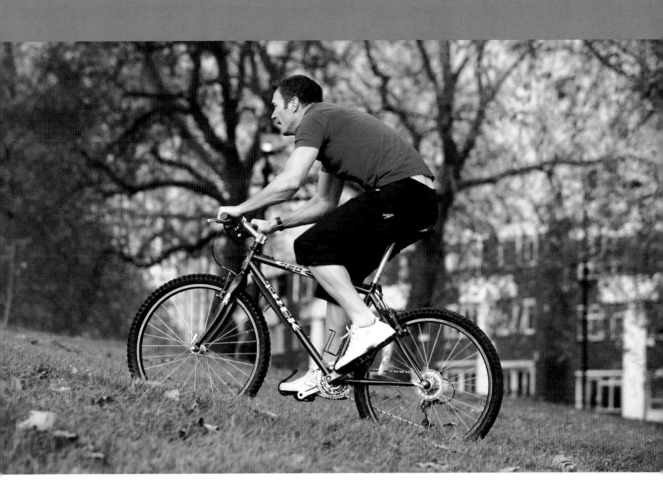

and improve your chances of maintaining your exercise programme in the long term, it's worth building in plenty of variety when designing your 30-minute workouts.

How do I make my workouts varied?

There is a number of ways to add variety to your 30-minute workouts. Here are my suggestions for a more interesting workout:

Use more than one type of exercise

There is no need to perform the same exercise for the entire 30-minute workout. To keep things interesting, divide the time between any or all of your chosen types of exercise: for example, try 10 minutes' walking, 10 minutes' jogging, 10 minutes' cycling.

Use different environments

The quickest way to boredom is to use the same walking, jogging or cycling route. Instead, you should continually vary the route. Use different environments to give you something new to look at while you exercise: the countryside, your immediate neighbourhood, a city centre. As well as choosing different environments, vary the type of route to include up and down hills, flat routes and undulating routes.

Use different techniques

Trying different techniques will add interest to your workout. For example, Nordic walking (using poles) and power walking (using your arms) can increase the intensity without changing the speed. If you swim, use different strokes to alter the intensity: front crawl is harder than breast stroke and butterfly is much harder than front crawl.

Use different intensities

Varying the intensity of exercise over the 30-minute workout is a further way to reduce boredom and it often increases the benefits gained from the workout. Try the following:

• **Negative split** Divide your session into two 15-minute blocks and make the second one harder than the first. Similarly you could divide the workout into three 10-minute blocks using different exercises and make each block progressively harder.

• **Speed play (sometimes termed Fartlek)** Within your 30 minutes of continuous exercise use short periods of medium- or hard-intensity effort interspersed with periods of easy exercise. For example, alternate 1 minute hard followed by 1 minute easy exercise for your 30 minutes. Alternatively, try 5 minutes at a medium intensity, 5 minutes easy, 10 minutes medium and end with 10 minutes easy. Choose any combination to make your total 30 minutes of exercise.

• **Intervals** Divide your workout into periods of activity, usually medium or hard intensity, interspersed with periods of rest. Try, for example, ten 2-minute bouts at a moderate intensity with a 1-minute rest between each bout. Alternatively, try twenty 30-second efforts at a hard intensity with a 1-minute recovery between efforts.

What does moderate intensity mean?

Intensity is simply a measure of how hard you are exercising. Because we are aiming to achieve 30 minutes of continuous exercise the intensity is usually termed 'moderate' or medium – meaning that it is an intensity that can be sustained without reducing the work load for the entire 30 minutes. Selecting an intensity that you can sustain for 30 minutes is often termed 'pacing'. Being able to pace yourself, or set your own intensity, can be very difficult if you are just taking up exercise or trying a new exercise. Starting too hard and being unable to finish the exercise is a common problem: ask a child to run around a track four times and you will see how hard it is to get this right. They always start off too quickly and are unable to complete the four laps without slowing down or stopping. With simple instruction and some practice, however, they will be able to control their pace and complete the four laps at a steady pace.

Start your exercise at an easy intensity and, over a number of workouts, increase the intensity as you become more experienced until you reach a moderate intensity that you can sustain for 30 minutes. Studies have shown that gradually increasing your intensity in this way lessens your chances of developing a medical problem because you are learning how your body responds to exercise and enhancing your enjoyment while building up to an increased activity level. Being able to measure at what intensity you are exercising is crucial for optimising your workout. It is important to understand what your target intensity is, how to assess what intensity you are working at and structure your programme accordingly.

While the health recommendations suggest moderate-intensity exercise, feel free to include easy- and hard-intensity bouts of exercise in your 30-minute workouts.

How do I measure intensity?

There are different ways to measure intensity during exercise, some more complex and technical than others. The most common and practical measures include psychological (how you feel) and physiological (how your body is responding) factors. There is no right or wrong method – choose the one that works for you.

Psychological measures for monitoring intensity

Psychological techniques use your own perception of how hard the exercise feels to set exercise intensity. One of the simplest and most widely used techniques is termed rating of perceived exertion (RPE). This approach uses your ability to detect and interpret sensations from your own body. In other words, you are monitoring how you feel and using that information to control how hard you are working. The great advantage of this method is that it uses feedback from multiple body systems that are then interpreted by the brain to give an overall feeling of effort.

Different scales are used to monitor RPE. The original technique uses a 15-point scale from 6 to 20 (above right), which is based upon heart rate. However, this method of estimating heart-rate response is valuable only for middle-aged men, so simpler scales are also used, including the modified 10-point scale (see right).

Rating of perceived exertion (Borg 15-point RPE scale)

6	No exertion at all
7	Extremely light
8	
9	Very light
10	
11	Light
12	
13	Somewhat hard
14	
15	Hard (heavy)
16	
17	Very hard
18	
19	Extremely hard
20	Maximum exertion

Modified rating of perceived exertion (RPE)

1	Resting
2	
3	Very easy
4	Easy
5	
6	Medium
7	
8	Hard
9	
10	Maximum

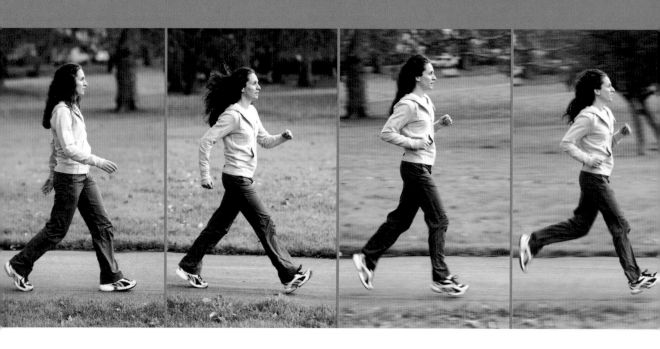

By learning to grade how you feel during exercise you can control the intensity without the need for technical equipment. To use an RPE scale optimally it is important to be able to anchor the bottom and the top of the scale. This means that the bottom of the scale is how you feel when you are sitting watching TV and the top of the scale is the hardest you have ever exercised. You can use RPE to rate the feeling of your whole body or certain areas only, such as your legs or arms. By choosing which areas you use to rate the intensity of exercise you can control the exercise, targeting certain parts of your body.

The more you use RPE to monitor and control intensity, the easier it becomes. For the first-time exerciser RPE is an excellent way to ensure you are working at the right intensity and you learn how to listen to your body. After a while you will not need to look at the RPE scale to know what intensity you are working at, which makes it the simplest of intensity-monitoring tools.

Physiological measures for monitoring intensity

Physiological measures use information from the response of your body, such as heart rate, or from how you are performing – for example, speed or number of steps or lengths – to give you information on how hard you are working. These rules of thumb are a guide to the intensity of exercise you are working at:

• Easy exercise is performed at an intensity that allows you to hold a full conversation while exercising

• Moderate exercise is performed at an intensity that allows you to converse in broken sentences and words while exercising

• Hard exercise is performed at an intensity that allows you to converse only in single words while exercising

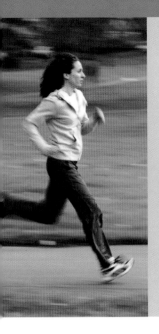

Walking and running pace descriptions

Rating of pace	Actual speed			
	mph	kph	minutes per mile	minutes per kilometre
Strolling	2–3	3–5	25–19.5	20–12
Brisk walking	3.5–4	5.5–7	17.5–13.5	11–8.5
Easy jogging	4.5–5	7.5–8	13–12	8–7.5
Medium jogging (easy running)	5.5–6	8.5–10	11.5–9.5	7–6
Running	6.5+	10.5+	9+	5.5+

Using speed to monitor intensity

The faster you go, the harder you have to work, therefore the higher the intensity. By calculating your speed you can monitor your intensity. The easiest way to use speed to monitor intensity is simply to time yourself around a certain route or over a known distance to give your baseline time. To increase the intensity on subsequent occasions, simply speed up to complete the same circuit in reduced time. A way to increase your pace evenly around the circuit is to pick some landmarks and make a mental note of how long it takes you to reach them. If you then ensure you arrive at each landmark ahead of your baseline time by the same amount for each one, you can achieve even pacing.

The table above gives you an idea of the average speed of various intensities of walking, jogging and running. In general walking is a lower-intensity exercise than jogging and jogging is a lower-intensity

exercise than running. However, you can increase your walking to a greater intensity than that of jogging by opting for power walking or Nordic walking. Both techniques help to reduce the impact on joints while increasing the overall benefit of the exercise.

For swimming, speed is the best way to monitor intensity. You can monitor your speed simply by increasing the number of lengths you swim in 30 minutes or you can use some of the ways of varying the effort outlined on page 170, such as negative splits, speed play and intervals, to change intensity. Swimming more lengths during your higher-intensity bouts of exercise will increase your intensity.

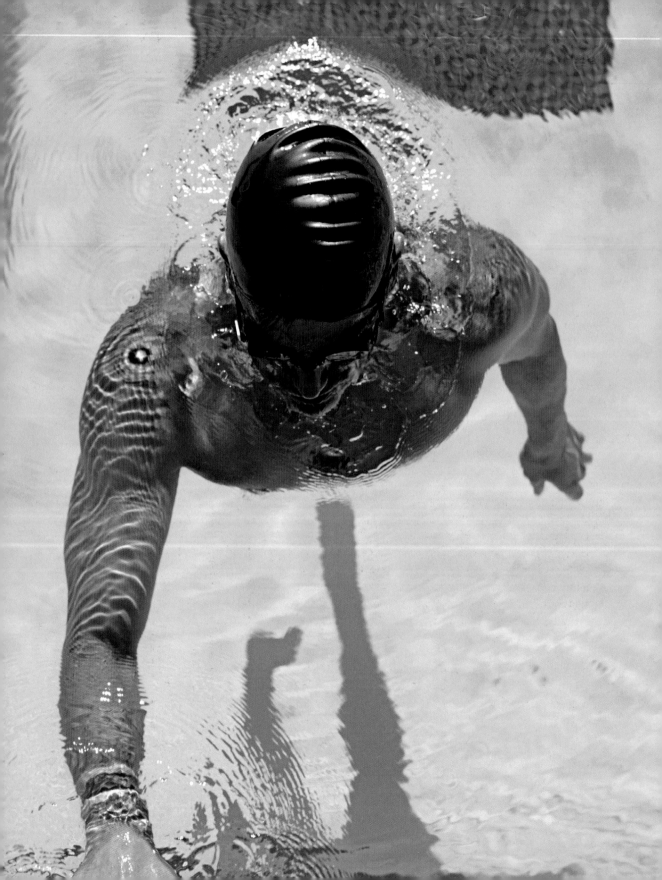

Using heart rate to monitor intensity

Heart rate is a measure of the number of times a minute your heart beats to pump blood around your body. During exercise you need to pump more blood around the body to provide the muscles with the oxygen and nutrients they need. We can use heart rate as a measure of the intensity of exercise because the harder you exercise, the higher the heart rate. As we get older our maximum heart rate decreases (by 1 beat per year on average – the same for men and women). This linear relationship allows us to use age to predict our maximum heart rate.

A very simple equation has been devised to estimate maximum heart rate:

$$\text{maximum heart rate} = 220 - \text{age}$$

For example, the maximum heart rate of a 40-year-old is:

$$220 - 40 = 180 \text{ beats per minute}$$

However, recent studies have shown that maximum heart rate may vary by as much as 20 beats from this estimate, so it can only be a rough guide. A more meaningful method is to calculate your target heart rate.

Target heart rates are based upon percentages of your maximum heart rate. In line with our use of easy-, medium- and hard-intensity exercise, heart-rate targets are 60 per cent, 70 per cent and 80 per cent respectively of maximum heart rate.

There is a simple equation to calculate the desired target heart rate:

$$\text{target heart rate} =$$
$$(220 - \text{age}) \times \text{target (60\%, 70\% or 80\%)}$$

For example, if a 50-year-old man wants to calculate his medium-intensity target heart rate, the equation is:

$$\text{target heart rate} =$$
$$(220 - 50) \times 0.7 = 119 \text{ beats per minute}$$

You can also use the table below to identify your target heart rate.

Target heart rate based on age using 220 – age

Age	Easy	Medium	Hard
20	120	140	160
25	117	137	156
30	114	133	152
35	111	130	148
40	108	126	144
45	105	123	140
50	102	119	136
55	99	116	132
60	96	112	128
65	93	109	124
70	90	105	120
75	87	102	116
80	84	98	112

Using resting heart rate can improve the prediction of your target heart rate. This method employs what is known as the Karvonen equation:

target heart rate = [(220 − age − resting heart rate) x target (60%, 70% or 80%)] + resting heart rate

If, for instance, a 40-year-old woman with a resting heart rate of 70 beats per minute wants to calculate her hard-intensity target heart rate, the calculation is:

target heart rate =
[(220 − 40 − 70) x 0.8] + 70 =
158 beats per minute

Target heart rate using your resting heart rate (Karvonen equation)

Resting heart rate	Age 20			Age 25			Age 30			Age 35		
	Easy	Medium	Hard	Easy	Medium	Hard	Easy	Medium	Hard	Easy	Medium	Hard
40	136	152	168	133	149	164	130	145	160	127	142	156
45	138	154	169	135	150	165	132	147	161	129	143	157
50	140	155	170	137	152	166	134	148	162	131	145	158
55	142	157	171	139	153	167	136	150	163	133	146	159
60	144	158	172	141	155	168	138	151	164	135	148	160
65	146	160	173	143	156	169	140	153	165	137	149	161
70	148	161	174	145	158	170	142	154	166	139	151	162
75	150	163	175	147	159	171	144	156	167	141	152	163
80	152	164	176	149	161	172	146	157	168	143	154	164
85	154	166	177	151	162	173	148	159	169	145	155	165
90	156	167	178	153	164	174	150	160	170	147	157	166

Resting heart rate	Age 40			Age 45			Age 50			Age 55		
	Easy	Medium	Hard	Easy	Medium	Hard	Easy	Medium	Hard	Easy	Medium	Hard
40	124	138	152	121	135	148	118	131	144	115	128	140
45	126	140	153	123	136	149	120	133	145	117	129	141
50	128	141	154	125	138	150	122	134	146	119	131	142
55	130	143	155	127	139	151	124	136	147	121	132	143
60	132	144	156	129	141	152	126	137	148	123	134	144
65	134	146	157	131	142	153	128	139	149	125	138	145
70	136	147	158	133	144	154	130	140	150	127	137	146
75	138	149	159	135	145	155	132	142	151	129	138	147
80	140	150	160	137	147	156	134	143	152	131	140	148
85	142	152	161	139	148	157	136	145	153	133	141	149
90	144	153	162	141	150	158	138	146	154	135	143	150

Alternatively, use the table below, based on the Karvonen equation, to predict your target heart rate taking into account your resting heart rate.

Resting heart rate	Age 60			Age 65			Age 70		
	Easy	Medium	Hard	Easy	Medium	Hard	Easy	Medium	Hard
40	112	124	136	109	121	132	106	117	128
45	114	126	137	111	122	133	108	129	129
50	116	127	138	113	124	134	110	120	130
55	118	129	139	115	125	135	112	122	131
60	120	130	140	117	127	136	114	123	132
65	122	132	141	119	128	137	116	125	133
70	124	133	142	121	130	138	118	126	134
75	126	135	143	123	131	139	120	128	135
80	128	136	144	125	133	140	122	129	136
85	130	138	145	127	134	141	124	131	137
90	132	139	146	129	136	142	126	132	138

Resting heart rate	Age 75			Age 80		
	Easy	Medium	Hard	Easy	Medium	Hard
40	103	114	124	100	110	120
45	105	115	125	102	112	121
50	107	117	126	104	113	122
55	109	118	127	106	115	123
60	111	120	128	108	116	124
65	113	121	129	110	118	125
70	115	123	130	112	119	126
75	117	124	131	114	121	127
80	119	126	132	116	122	128
85	121	127	133	118	124	129
90	123	129	134	120	125	130

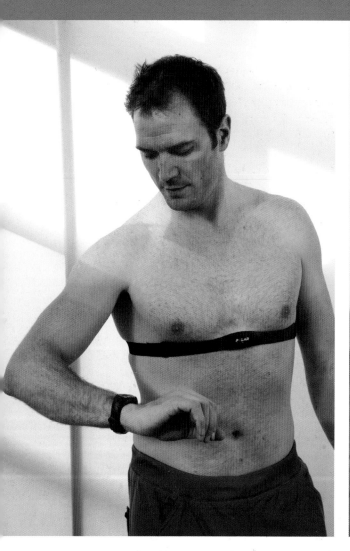

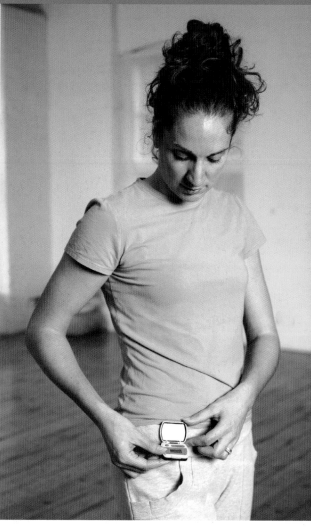

Heart-rate monitors The easiest way to measure heart rate during exercise is to use a heart-rate monitor. Heart-rate monitors are simple to use and inexpensive to buy. Most strap around your chest to pick up signals from your heart and transmit them to a wrist watch. They give instantaneous feedback on how hard you are working.

Using pedometers to monitor intensity
A pedometer is a device about the size of a matchbox that can be attached to your belt or trouser top. It records the number of steps you take during walking, jogging or running (it is not helpful for other forms of exercise). A pedometer is a cheap and very useful tool for estimating your physical activity levels. You can use the step index on page 179 to identify your activity category.

The step index to estimate your activity level

Steps per day	Activity level
up to 5,000	Very low
5,000–7,500	Low
7,500–10,000	Moderate
10,000–12,500	Active
12,500+	Very active

The target number of steps per day recommended by government officials is 10,000. This may sound like a huge total but the figure is based on the average number of steps taken during a 30-minute walk (try it and you'll see!). You can use the 10,000 steps per day as your goal, if necessary, depending on your activity level: set yourself short-term targets and increase your steps per day by a small number (around 500 steps) each week to build up to 10,000 steps per day. You could always set your target as a weekly total, allowing yourself the flexibility to increase the number of steps when you feel ready and when the weather is good enough – because forcing yourself to walk, jog or run in poor weather is no fun and will not help you maintain your exercise programme.

Take every opportunity to increase the number of steps you take in a day. You don't have to incorporate dedicated walks into your routine – just try some of these easy ways to bring up the total:

• Take the stairs rather than the lift

• Park your car as far away from where you are going as reasonably possible

• Walk the long way around the office

• Take short walking breaks from your desk

Pedometers can also be very valuable in measuring intensity of exercise. First determine the number of steps you take during a normal walk. Use this baseline number of steps as your target for every walk of the same duration and try to increase the number of steps you take whenever you go for a walk. For improved accuracy in measuring intensity, divide the duration of the walk (in minutes) by the number of steps to calculate the number of steps per minute. That baseline step rate per minute then becomes the target to beat when you are out walking. Checking your step rate regularly will help you maintain the same intensity. Moving from walking to jogging to running automatically increases your intensity. When you start jogging or running recalculate the number of steps as described above and set yourself new targets.

8

Weekly training programmes

Progressive programme

If you are taking up exercise for the first time or returning to it after a long period of inactivity it is important to remember the lessons learned in earlier chapters. Before starting your exercise programme, go back to Chapter 3 and answer the questions contained in the 'starting exercise for the first time' box (see page 31). Having established whether you need to see your GP first and take advice if necessary, you can begin your exercise programme. It is important to build progressive overload (see page 23) into your programme.

The following five programmes constitute an example of a 15-week programme that takes you from zero to 150 minutes. Each programme is of three weeks' duration and the idea is to increase the intensity of each session week by week, starting with easy in week 1, moving to medium in week 2 and finally to hard in the third week of the programme. If you are struggling to achieve the weekly programme, simply extend the programme for a week or two to allow yourself to adapt fully before moving on.

You can start a programme on any day of the week, but the key thing is to follow the days in the order I've set them so that the intensity of your workouts is balanced across the week.

Weeks 1–3: 30 minutes

DAY 1	DAY 2	DAY 3	DAY 4
5-minute workout **Flexibility:** • Upper calf • Hamstring – standing • Lower back • Upper back • Biceps • Neck stretch	**5-minute workout** **Strength and power:** • Squat • Push-up • Static running	Rest day	**10-minute workout** • Walk

DAY 5	DAY 6	DAY 7
Rest day	Rest day	**10-minute workout** • 3-minute walk • 1-minute skip • 1-minute stair climb **repeat once**

Weeks 4–6: 60 minutes

DAY 1	DAY 2	DAY 3	DAY 4
5-minute workout **Flexibility:** • Triceps • Upper body stretch • Groin • Seated outer thigh • Hamstring – seated • Lower calf	**30-minute workout** • Walk	**10-minute workout** • 2-minute walk • 2-minute skip • 2-minute walk • 2-minute skip • 2-minute walk	Rest day

DAY 5	DAY 6	DAY 7
10-minute workout • 1-minute skip • Push-up • Abdominal curl • Jump squat • Abdominal curl with twist • 1-minute skip	**5-minute workout** **Strength and power:** • Jump squat • Static running • Push-up	Rest day

Weeks 7–9: 90 minutes

DAY 1

5-minute workout **Flexibility:** • Hamstring – seated • Thigh • Lower back • Triceps • Biceps • Side neck	**5-minute workout** **Strength and power:** • Squat • Push-up • Abdominal curl • Side lunge

DAY 2

30-minute workout
• Swim

DAY 3

10-minute workout
• 2-minute skip
• 3-minute walk
repeat twice

DAY 4

Rest day

DAY 5

5-minute workout **Core strength and stability:** • Plank • Toe touch • Side raise • Leg pull	**5-minute workout** **Band exercises:** • Shoulder press • Bent-over rowing • Sumo squat

DAY 6

30-minute workout
• 5-minute easy walk
• 3-minute medium walk
• 2-minute jog
repeat 3 times

DAY 7

Rest day

Weeks 10–12: 120 minutes

DAY 1

5-minute workout **Flexibility:** • Lower calf • Hamstring – seated • Thigh • Lower back • Upper back • Chest • Side neck	**5-minute workout** **Strength and power:** • Squat • Push-up • Lunge	**5-minute workout** **Core strength and stability:** • Lower back and core • Leg lower • Shoulder bridge	**5-minute workout** **Band exercises:** • Clean • Bicep curl • Shoulder press

DAY 2

30-minute workout
• 3-minute easy walk
• 2-minute medium walk
• 1-minute jog
repeat 5 times

10-minute workout
• 2-minute skip
• Jump squat
• Push-up
• Lunge
• Abdominal curl
• 2-minute skip

DAY 3

5-minute workout **Strength and power:** • Calf raise • Push-up • Lunge	**10-minute workout** • Squat (Strength and power) • Abdominal curl • Calf raise • Abdominal curl with twist • Lunge • Push-up • Jump squat

Weeks 10–12: 120 minutes (cont.)

DAY 4	DAY 5	DAY 6	DAY 7
10-minute workout • 5-minute skip • 3-minute walk • 2-minute jog	**5-minute workout** **Bum, tum and thighs:** • Bum lift • Oyster • Cushion squeeze	**30-minute workout** Swim: • 10-minute easy to medium • 10 x (2 lengths hard, 30 seconds rest) • 10-minute easy to medium	Rest day

Weeks 13–15: 150 minutes

DAY 1

5-minute workout **Flexibility:** • Upper calf • Upper back • Hamstring – standing • Hips – Z-stretch • Neck extension • Neck flexion	**5-minute workout** **Core strength and stability:** • Plank • Toe touch • Lower back and core	**5-minute workout** **Bum, tum and thighs:** • Sumo • Cushion squeeze • Side lift	**5-minute workout** **Band exercises:** • Clean • Leg extension • Leg curl

DAY 1 (cont.)	DAY 2	DAY 3	
10-minute workout • 1-minute skip • 1-minute walk • 1-minute stair climb • 1-minute walk • 1-minute jog repeat once	**30-minute workout** • 10-minute easy walk • 5 x (1-minute hill walk with a walk down to the start) • 10-minute easy walk	**10-minute workout** **Band exercises:** • Squat • Leg extension • Bicep curl • Leg curl • Tricep curl • Clean • Bent-over rowing	**5-minute workout** **Band exercises:** • Bent-over rowing • Shoulder press • Bicep curl

DAY 4	DAY 5		DAY 6
30-minute workout • Swim	**5-minute workout** **Flexibility:** • Lower calf • Bum • Camel • Neck stretch • Chest • Triceps • Biceps	**10-minute workout** • Sumo • Push-up • Jump squat • Abdominal curl • Calf raise • Static running • Lunge	**30-minute workout** • Cycle (hilly route) **DAY 7** Rest day

Back pain affects a huge number of people and negatively impacts on their overall quality of life. Poor fitness in the form of strength, strength endurance and flexibility are amongst the major causes of low back pain. The lower-back pain programme is an example of the sort of programme you can use to improve those key areas leading to back pain.

This programme is at an easy intensity and is ideal for those who are not currently physically active. Remember always to work within the limits of pain – stop when it hurts!

Lower-back-pain programme (easy)

DAY 1			
5-minute workout Flexibility: • Lower back • Hamstring – seated • Bum and hip • Inner thigh • Lower back and hips	**5-minute workout Core strength and stability:** • Lower back and core • Plank • Cat	**5-minute workout Bum, tum and thighs:** • Bum lift • Sumo • Cushion squeeze	**10-minute workout** • 2-minute easy walk • 3 x (1-minute hard walk, 1-minute easy walk) • 2-minute easy walk

DAY 2	DAY 3		
30-minute workout • 5-minute easy walk • 5-minute medium walk **repeat 3 times**	**5-minute workout Strength and power:** • Push-up • Abdominal curl • Lunge	**5-minute workout Core strength and stability:** • Leg pull • Shoulder bridge • Toe touch	**10-minute workout** • 3-minute stair climb • Push-up • Static running • Tricep curl • 3-minute stair climb

DAY 4	DAY 5		
30-minute workout • Swim: alternating strokes (easy to medium)	**5-minute workout Flexibility:** • Seated outer thigh • Groin • Hip • Hip flexor • Lower back • Upper back • Chest • Neck stretch	**5-minute workout Core strength and stability:** • Toe touch • Cat • Side raise • Plank	**5-minute workout Strength and power:** • Squat • Abdominal curl with twist • Side lunge

DAY 6	DAY 7
30-minute workout • Cycle (easy)	Rest day

Skiing is a great form of exercise but unfortunately it is one of the most injury-prone sports, particularly for poorly conditioned people with low levels of cardiovascular fitness and strength. Improving your overall fitness is key to reducing the possibility of injury and increasing your enjoyment on the slopes. This programme is designed to improve all those areas of cardiovascular fitness, strength, strength endurance and flexibility that reduce the likelihood of claiming on your insurance!

Skiing programme (hard)

DAY 1

5-minute workout **Flexibility:**	**5-minute workout** **Core strength and stability:**	**5-minute workout** **Strength and power:**	**5-minute workout** **Band exercises:**
• Hip flexor • Lower back • Bum • Bum and hip • Hip • Groin	• Plank • Leg lower • Upright stability	• Calf raise • Squat • Static running • Push-up	• Bicep curl • Shoulder press • Tricep curl

DAY 1 (cont.)	DAY 2	DAY 3	
10-minute workout • 3-minute skip • Jump squat • Push-up • Static running • 3-minute skip	**30-minute workout** • 5-minute medium walk • 10 x (1-minute hard walk, 1-minute easy walk) • 5-minute medium-to-easy walk	**10-minute workout** • 2-minute medium run • 6 x (30-second hard run, 30-second walk) • 2-minute easy-to-medium run	**5-minute workout** **Bum, tum and thighs:** • Sumo • Leg raise • Cushion squeeze

DAY 3 (cont.)	DAY 4	DAY 5	
5-minute workout **Strength and power:** • Jump squat • Lunge • Push-up	**30-minute workout** • Swim	**5-minute workout** **Flexibility:** • Upper calf • Thigh • Inner thigh • Seated outer thigh • Hamstring • Lower back and hips	**10-minute workout** • 1-minute stair climb • Lunge • Abdominal curl • 1-minute stair climb • Toe touch • Side lunge • 1-minute stair climb

DAY 5 (cont.)	DAY 6	DAY 7
5-minute workout **Band exercises:** • Leg extension • Leg curl • Squat	**30-minute workout** • 10 minute easy-to-medium cycle • 5 x (1-minute hill climb (hard) with a free-wheel back to the start) • 5-minute easy-to-medium cycle	Rest day

Upper-body strength is important for all sorts of reasons: maintaining muscle mass as we get older, improving our ability to perform daily tasks, improving athletic performance and simply looking good on the beach. The upper-body-strength programme is an example of how to focus your sessions on one particular area of the body.

The programme here is a hard intensity one that is perfect for improving athletic performance and looking good. By simply adapting the exercises and intensity you can use these sessions for a range of goals. By focusing on small areas of the body for short periods of time you can increase motivation and target short-term goals. A change is as good as rest!

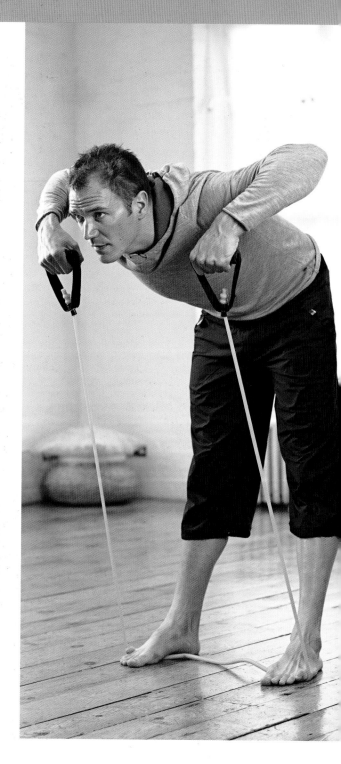

Upper-body-strength programme (hard)

DAY 1

5-minute workout Flexibility:	5-minute workout Strength and power:	5-minute workout Band exercises:	5-minute workout Band exercises:
• Neck flexion • Neck extension • Side neck • Upper back • Triceps • Back of shoulder	• Push-up • Abdominal curl • Neck-up	• Shoulder press • Anterior deltoid • Posterior deltoid	• Clean • Tricep curl • Bicep curl

DAY 1 (cont.)	DAY 2	DAY 3	
10-minute workout • Nordic walk (hard)	30-minute workout Swim: • 5 minutes easy • 3 minutes medium • 2 minutes hard repeat 3 times	10-minute workout • Plank • Abdominal curl • Shoulder bridge • Leg pull • Abdominal curl with twist • Lower back and core • Push-up	5-minute workout Strength and power/ Band exercises: • Push-up • Clean • Shoulder press

DAY 3 (cont.)	DAY 4		DAY 5
5-minute workout Core strength and stability: • Lower back and core • Plank • Toe touch	30-minute workout Swim: • 5 minutes easy • 10 x (2 lengths hard, 1-minute recovery) • 5 minutes easy	• 10 x (1 length hard, 30-second recovery) • 5 minutes easy • 5 x (1 length butterfly, 30-second recovery)	5-minute workout Flexibility: • Lower back • Biceps • Upper body • Lower back and hips • Camel • Chest

DAY 5		DAY 6	
10-minute workout: • Push-up • Tricep curl • Abdominal curl • Neck-up • Abdominal curl with twist • Push-up	5-minute workout Band exercises: • Clean • Tricep curl • Bicep curl	10-minute workout Band exercises: • Clean • Shoulder press • Tricep curl • Bicep curl • Anterior deltoid • Bent-over rowing	5-minute workout Band exercises: • Anterior deltoid • Medial deltoid • Posterior deltoid • Shoulder press

DAY 6 (cont.)	DAY 7
5-minute workout Core strength and stability: • Cat • Leg pull • Shoulder bridge	Rest day

As we age **bone mineral density** begins to fall. This is particularly true for women following the menopause. Exercises that increase the loading (e.g. jumping, skipping) and twisting forces on the bone are important for two reasons. First, as a pre-menopausal woman you can maximise your bone mineral density and, second, you can reduce – even halt – the rate of bone mineral loss in later life.

This programme is a simple way to maintain and improve bone mineral density and it's good for women and men of all ages.

Bone-health programme (medium)

DAY 1

5-minute workout **Flexibility:**	5-minute workout **Strength and power:**	5-minute workout **Band exercises:**	5-minute workout **Band exercises:**
• Lower back • Seated outer thigh • Upper back • Hamstring – seated • Neck stretch • Chest	• Squat • Static run • Jump squat	• Anterior deltoid • Shoulder press • Bent-over rowing	• Clean • Leg extension • Leg curl

DAY 1 (cont.)	DAY 2	DAY 3	
10-minute workout • 10-minute skip	30-minute workout • 5-minute easy walk • 5-minute medium walk • 5-minute hard walk **repeat twice**	10-minute workout • 3-minute skip • Squat (Strength and power) • Push-up • Jump squat • 3-minute skip	5-minute workout **Core strength and stability:** • Toe touch • Upright stability • Leg pull

DAY 4	DAY 5		DAY 6
30-minute workout • Hill walking (Nordic walking with poles if possible)	5-minute workout **Strength and power:** • Push-up • Neck-up • Jump squat	10-minute workout • 2-minute skip • 2-minute stair climb • 2-minute skip • 2-minute stair climb • 2-minute skip	30-minute workout • 5-minute easy walk • 5-minute cycle • 5-minute jog **repeat twice**

DAY 7
Rest day

The most common and most visible areas of the body where we deposit fat are the **bum, tummy and thighs.** Most people use dieting alone to reduce the fat deposits here although they are notoriously difficult areas to shift fat from. Even if we manage to lose some of it through dieting, without muscular strength and tone we have no shape (curve appeal).

The following programme is an example of how you can target these difficult-to-reach areas and improve your aesthetic quality by enhancing your overall shape.

Bum, tum and thighs programme (medium)

DAY 1

5-minute workout **Flexibility:**	**5-minute workout** **Strength and power:**	**5-minute workout** **Bum, tum and thighs:**	**5-minute workout** **Core strength and stability:**
• Hamstring – seated • Seated outer thigh • Hip flexor • Groin • Bum • Bum and hip	• Squat • Side lunge • Abdominal curl	• Bum lift • Oyster • Cushion squeeze	• Toe touch • Plank • Abdominal curl with twist

DAY 2 / DAY 3

30-minute workout	**10-minute workout**	**5-minute workout** **Bum, tum and thighs:**	**5-minute workout** **Strength and power:**
• 5-minute easy walk • 10 x (1-minute hard walk, 1-minute easy walk) • 5-minute easy walk	• 1-minute stair climb • 1-minute skip • Squat (Strength and power) • Sumo • Jump squat • 1-minute skip • 1-minute stair climb	• Leg raise • Side lift • Sumo	• Static running • Lunge • Abdominal curl

DAY 4 / DAY 5

30-minute workout	**5-minute workout** **Flexibility:**	**10-minute workout**	**5-minute workout** **Band exercises:**
• 5-minute easy-to-medium cycle • 10 x (1-minute hill climb with a free-wheel back to the start) • 5-minute easy cycle	• Hamstring – standing • Hips – Z-stretch • Camel • Bum • Inner thigh	• Abdominal curl • Abdominal curl with twist • Squat (Strength and power) • Tricep curl • Lunge • Static running • Lower back and core	• Leg extension • Outer thigh • Sumo squat

DAY 6 / DAY 7

30-minute workout	DAY 7
• 10-minute easy-to-medium walk • 5 x (1-minute hill walk with easy walk down to the start) • 10-minute easy walk	Rest day

Index

Acknowledgements

I would like to thank Muna Reyal for her initial interest and encouragement, and the whole team at Kyle Cathie for their unwavering support and for believing in the concept of this book from the start. In particular I would like to thank Jenny Wheatley for her wonderfully relaxed approach and invaluable feedback and advice on all aspects of the book. Thanks also to Debbie Catchpole for making the project a reality.

Thanks go to my models: Tony Gibb, Peter Slater, Laura Wheatley and my wife Penny, whose eternal support in all areas of my life is immeasurable. Thanks also to my daughter, Maya, who kept us amused during our long shoots!

I would like to thank Stephanie Evans for making sense of my manuscript, and Alison Fenton for doing such a superb job of designing the book.

The terrific clothing was supplied by Speedo and Howies. Thanks to them for their generosity in this and other projects.

A very special thanks to Tony Chau for his fantastic photography. Tony managed to make exercise come to life in a way that shows unique skill.

Finally, I would like to thank my Mum and Dad, George and Peggy, who have made me what I am.

Photographic acknowledgements

All photography by Tony Chau except for the following:

Page 2 Pixland / Corbis
Page 4 Courtesy of *This Morning*
Pages 6 –7 Victoria Dawe
Page 11 Aflo Foto Agency / Alamy
Page 15 Stockbyte / Alamy
Page 19 JUPITERIMAGES / BananaStock / Alamy
Page 21 Redfx / Alamy
Page 23 Mary-Ella Keith / Alamy
Page 27 Bloomimage / Corbis
Page 28 Stockbyte / Alamy
Page 30 PhotoAlto / Alamy
Page 37 Peter Fakler / Alamy
Page 164 Andrew O'Toole / Zefa / Corbis
Page 165 Image Source Black / Alamy
Page 174 Photodisc / Alamy